understand pain.

take back control.

A PRACTICAL GUIDE TO CHRONIC PAIN MANAGEMENT

DAVID WALTON

Published in the UK
in 2019 by Icon Books Ltd,
Omnibus Business Centre,
39–41 North Road,
London N7 9DP
email: info@iconbooks.com
www.iconbooks.com

Sold in the UK, Europe and Asia
by Faber & Faber Ltd,
Bloomsbury House,
74–77 Great Russell Street,
London WC1B 3DA
or their agents

Distributed in the UK,
Europe and Asia
by Grantham Book Services,
Trent Road, Grantham NG31 7XQ

Distributed in South Africa
by Jonathan Ball,
Office B4, The District,
41 Sir Lowry Road,
Woodstock 7925

Distributed in India
by Penguin Books India,
7th Floor, Infinity Tower –
C, DLF Cyber City,
Gurgaon 122002, Haryana

Distributed in Australia and
New Zealand
by Allen & Unwin Pty Ltd,
PO Box 8500,
83 Alexander Street,
Crows Nest,
NSW 2065

Distributed in Canada
by Publishers Group Canada,
76 Stafford Street, Unit 300,
Toronto,
Ontario M6J 2S1

Distributed in the USA
by Publishers Group West,
1700 Fourth Street,
Berkeley, CA 94710

ISBN: 978-178578-449-1

Typeset in Avenir by Marie Doherty

Printed and bound in Great Britain
by Clays Ltd, Elcograf S.p.A.

About Self-management

Pain is not pleasant. It hurts. But many chronic pain patients attending pain clinics say the real problem isn't the amount of pain as such. It's how pain weaves its way into their everyday lives, limiting activity and preventing any sense of being in control that they find most exhausting. And, sometimes, overwhelming.

There are many different causes of long-term pain, and we do not know them all yet. But whether you suffer chronic pain yourself, or are supporting someone else who does, managing it effectively requires the person who experiences it to become their own 'pain manager'. This means getting to grips with a newly emerging understanding of how pain really works. Understanding how pain varies from one person to another is vital because, while there are many ways of coping, what works for one person may not for someone else, even with an identical condition.

The book uses recent research into pain management combined with real patient experiences to help you develop a personal pain management plan. It contains questionnaires, explanations and tools, and is intended to support you when having discussions with doctors or clinical advisers about your personal circumstances. The plan is the start of a journey, first and critically, to understand the pain and your body; then to take control of it, moving from passively enduring to exercising control and deciding how you want to live. Using what you learn, you can decide which of the practical ideas are best for you personally, and what help and support you may need, and you will discover how your understanding and outlook are really the key to overcoming your pain.

Note

The research and ideas described in the book come from many sources. Major contributions by individuals have been acknowledged, but it has not been possible to reference every idea, development or research conclusion. The author wishes to thank all those health and allied professionals whose work has underpinned this distillation of current thinking about pain management.

It is important to understand, however, that the contents of this book are of a general nature, based on the best information available to the author at the time of writing. The book does not constitute individual medical advice – so always consult a doctor or appropriate professional about your particular circumstances and condition. Neither the author nor the publisher shall be liable or responsible for any loss or damage allegedly arising from any information or suggestion in this book.

Contents

Biographical Note

Dr David Walton

David was initially trained as a cognitive and clinical psychologist in the UK's national health service (NHS). He subsequently qualified as an occupational psychologist, taking up an executive management post in public service. In 1988, he was appointed principal psychologist in the UN Research Institute for Social Development, working mainly on conflict resolution and institutional capacity building. He returned to health services and consultancy work in the UK, specialising in working with cancer patients, developing clinical teams and improving patient experiences.

He has worked with people with pain in the NHS and voluntary sectors, run hospital pain management clinics and researches developments in pain science. A member of the British Pain Society, he is particularly interested in increasing access to psychological services and their role in pain management and emotional distress.

Acknowledgements

Many people have helped turn the idea for this book into reality. Kiera, my Icon editor, did a magnificent job rescuing the book from being a barely readable medicalised tome. She improved it immeasurably. My experienced clinical reviewers (Beth and Tony, Chris and Alan, Ayesha, Mark and Austin) who contributed thoughts and ideas for the content and focus – and my family (Liz and Ros) for putting up with me as it was written. My thanks.

1. How Can You Use This Book?

Introduction

I have just come into my office from the garden, having enjoyed a few minutes in the all too rare Yorkshire sunshine. I had been contemplating the themes this book should cover when my wife Liz called to me, 'Just be careful. Don't do too much out there!'

Fifteen years ago, I had a serious riding accident, and everything changed. I have the aftermath of a spine fractured in five places, various hip and neck problems, osteoarthritis, diabetes and a knee which must be resurfaced, after the opposite hip gave way – it is currently awaiting replacement surgery. These, together with insomnia, fatigue and a possible cardiac condition, now give me the chronic pain which many people I have worked with in pain clinics suffer.

So, in calling out to me, Liz was generously expressing concern because I'm still wobbly on the crutches and she didn't want me to hurt myself. However, in those nine words she had encapsulated a significant problem for anyone trying to manage pain. It's great to have someone who cares. But as the butt of examinations, tests, operations and advice about health from every quarter, it can feel all too easy to descend into the role of a dependent 'patient', becoming reliant on medics and carers, giving away control, asking too few questions and reacting passively. It's almost inevitable when you are very ill, are unable to do much and the treatment is in the hands of professionals.

But for those of us with chronic pain where the conditions causing it cannot be easily cured, this outlook is problematic. When our thinking becomes passive, giving away control and 'ruminating' on our limitations and pain episodes, it creates changes in our nervous systems and body chemistry, paradoxically making pain *more* likely.

This view has been shaped by my work with brilliant researchers, colleagues and patients whose daily struggles have put my own pains completely in the shade. I have spent time with colleagues from the British Pain Society and International Association for the Study of Pain, who encourage research and collate the enormous amount of new knowledge on the subject. The emerging evidence about the role of psychological processes in 'nociception' – pain awareness and control – is particularly impressive, as are the experiences of chronic pain patients trying the resulting newly developed approaches.

This book draws upon pioneering work by, among others, neuroscientist Lorimer Moseley, clinical educationalist David Butler and psychologists Aaron Beck and Martin Seligman – supported by what I will call the neuroscience revolution, which shows that pain control owes much to the individual's understanding of how tissue injuries, the brain and our nervous systems work together. This is much more complex than 'the power of positive thinking alone'. As a practical introduction to this subject, the book will explore some of these exciting new ideas about pain management in (hopefully) a common-sense, non-clinical way.

Chronic pain, for those experiencing it, can be severe and disabling. World Health Organisation (WHO) data show it is an enormous health problem. Globally, it is estimated that as many as one in ten adult individuals are newly diagnosed with chronic pain each year. About one in five, or about 1.5 billion people, suffer from chronic pain, with prevalence increasing with age. Arthritis, post-operative, nerve damage and cancer pain are the leading causes. Reliable estimates indicate chronic pain prevalence at between 25 and 50 per cent in the US and Europe.

In the UK, recent statistics show that 43.5 per cent of the population experience chronic pain. Approximately 8 million people in the UK say their pain is severely disabling, and the Chief Medical Officer reports that 16 per cent of sufferers feel their pain is so bad that they sometimes want to die. As if that weren't bad enough, a quarter of joint pain sufferers lose their jobs, resulting in a poor quality of life. Studies show that lower back pain is ranked highest in terms of the burden of disease (out of 291 conditions). Four of the top twelve disabling conditions globally are persistent pain conditions.

Most people 'just get on with it' using over-the-counter or prescription drugs. Even with medication, the effects of chronic pain on quality of life are known to be highly damaging. A reported 41 per cent of people who attend UK pain clinics have been prevented from working by pain. Persistent pain also affects motivation, mental health and resilience, as well as the sufferer's family or carers. It can distort their lives, finances, living arrangements and relationships.

Global statistics about chronic pain show that its prevalence varies according to income levels and care facilities in that country. For example, the link between levels of pain, the economy and care systems in the UK recently led the Royal College of Anaesthetists' Faculty of Pain Medicine to acknowledge that economic considerations have put pain services at risk. Making the case for implementing agreed standards for pain diagnosis and treatment, they describe how pain can be all too easy to ignore, even by clinicians. This is because it is often seen as a non-life-threatening condition, so the clinical consequences of untreated pain are neither immediate nor prioritised. They report findings that pain is frequently under-addressed, under-managed and under-treated because of time and resource limitations. Startlingly, onward referral of patients with unresolved pain for more costly specialist care is also neglected.

But some progress is undoubtedly being made. Standards for pain management and services are becoming clearer, despite funding, staff, skills and time remaining in short supply. To cope, people with pain need to know what treatments and services are available and what they themselves can do to relieve it. That is where this book can help.

There are many guides and booklets about pain available already, which this book will complement, providing practical help with the challenge of taking control. Even with a supportive clinical team, coping with a painful condition requires skill, resilience and effective thinking skills, as well as decision making, planning and problem solving. Relationships with your doctors are important, so I hope the book will also enable you to have more effective discussions with them about your pain experience and how it can be controlled.

REMEMBER THIS!!! The book is organised into two parts:
The ideas which recent research suggests are critical to improving pain management are covered in **Part One**.

Part Two then looks at strategies and issues which chronic pain patients tell us have helped them to self-manage their pain.

Throughout the book there are questionnaires to measure your own situation, templates you can use and examples or case studies you may find useful.

Chapter 5 is especially important, exploring what you might need to include in a personal pain management plan. One aspect it covers is a 'Pain Management Wheel' which shows some of the options for pain control that we'll explore in Part Two. However, to fully understand what your plan for pain control could contain, wait until you have read all the remaining chapters in Part Two before you commit to your complete plan.

Experiences Coping with Pain

Over the last ten years, many people have found that really understanding their pain – knowing what influences it and recognising how their body and mind react to it – is profoundly helpful. Each person is individual and the circumstances they face are unique. However, understanding the circumstances other people face may offer some insights into coping with your own situation. What follows are real descriptions of how some pain sufferers' journeys began – presented in their own words. What do you make of their attitudes and reactions to their pain?

> **Person A** *is a no-nonsense, stoic individual, happy to get whatever medical advice is on offer and to act on it.*

❝ As a nurse, I have always been sensitive to people with pain – from injuries or from long-term conditions. I have always been pretty strong and maybe too busy in the hospital where I worked – so I cut corners. One day I fell and injured my hip and strained my shoulders and neck when I tried to get up. At first, I was prescribed a course of physiotherapy with an anti-inflammatory painkiller [naproxen] and the opioid co-codamol. The pain would ease temporarily and then return. It started when I woke – after little sleep – and built up the more I did anything through the day. I also had pain in both my hips, coccyx, left leg and foot.

I spent lots of money on physio and weekly Pilates classes after that and took the drugs I was prescribed, but my life still felt like it was on hold. I even cut down socialising with friends because sitting down was so uncomfortable.

Three years ago, I was prescribed injections of an anaesthetic and steroids into my spine. They gave me some relief, but not for long. Last year I was advised to have surgery, during which three of my vertebrae would be fused together with pins. Doctors are reluctant to carry out this type of surgery except as a last resort because it limits movement and adds pressure on the rest of the spine, possibly causing further problems, so I decided to have only two vertebrae done. It should have given me relief for years, but the pain's back and I just don't know what to do. They've given me Tramadol now and I take about eighteen other anti-inflammatory and nerve pain pills every day. 〟

Person B *is looking for an alternative treatment because she feels little progress is being made with conventional treatments.*

❝ I am 53 and was working as a disability carer and part-time gymnastic coach. I was very active when I was young, and I suppose I put my increasing stiffness and aches down to just getting older. I realised something more was involved when I had to lie back on the bed with my feet in the air to get my socks on. Stiffness was taking over my life, but I just thought, 'It's no fun getting older!'

I started to get severe pain four years ago and it became so bad I couldn't walk any more without help. My knees, ankles, wrists, elbows and shoulder joints were hot and inflamed. The hospital said it is rheumatoid arthritis, incurable … it's an autoimmune disorder where the body attacks its own cells, in this case the lining of my joints, producing chronic inflammation and eventually bone deformity. They have given me lots of medication including painkillers and something called methotrexate to damp down my immune system and block inflammatory proteins. The drugs stopped working earlier this year, so we're trying a cancer drug which targets my white blood cells. I'm supposed to be on it for life, but the pain just isn't going away. I've heard of something called vagal nerve stimulation that I'd like to try. **"**

These are the words of six people attending recent UK pain management workshops.

" • Pain changes you completely … It just takes your life away. Your whole personality changes.
 • It does affect your self-esteem because you always think about – well, I know they're negative thoughts really that you shouldn't have, but it's very difficult not to sometimes – you think about the things that you used to do and how you were a very sociable person.

- Pain is exhausting … You must walk slowly. You have to stop and make an excuse or pretend to look in a shop window so that you can put your hand on the window and rest a moment. It's humiliating.
- If I go somewhere I have to take a cushion because I can't tolerate a hard seat for any length of time. That, at my age, is embarrassing, because I'm comparatively young to have my body in this state.
- Pain is frustrating because you can't do things for yourself … Everything's a challenge.
- Pain is deep in my side and when it's really bad I'm not able to breathe deep, because when I breathe in deep it hurts.
- I get very depressed and anxious about it … it's frightening, especially when you live on your own.
- Pain can make you feel lonely because you feel that you're the only one who is suffering and can cope with it, and that is a lonely experience.
- I can't tie shoelaces now, so I've just got these slip-ons and a long shoehorn. You do make these adjustments as you go along.
- I can't keep my head down to read a book now so I put my book on a music stand. It works brilliantly.
- Thinking in advance. I'm planning my life out, pre-empting pain … I have a mattress behind my settee in my front room and I'll just have to lay that on the floor, in case I can't get up the stairs. **"**

Person C has a condition predominantly experienced by women and wants to find alternative treatments for it.

" I have been a sufferer of fibromyalgia for nearly three years now. The pain is constant and excruciating, but you can't really show that, can you? I've been hospitalised for weeks at a time (both in the UK and in the US), and I have seen three GPs and four consultants (neurologists and rheumatologists). I have been prescribed OxyNorm, OxyContin, Lyrica, Cymbalta, Savella, Amitriptyline and took part in a trial for a French drug call Ixel. Not one of these drugs helped decrease the pain I have, and the trial drug caused problems with my heart. The women in the clinic I go to now have really lost faith with doctors and so have I really. So, I am now going to a homeopathic practitioner and doing my own research. "

THINK ABOUT IT What conclusions do you draw from reading these stories? What impressions do you have of the people? How are they dealing with the situations they face? Jot down your thoughts in a notebook.

You will have seen from these stories that the circumstances which bring pain do something else too – they create a strong risk of our becoming dependent on anybody associated with healthcare because chronic pain makes us feel vulnerable and even hopeless. We think, 'They must know more than us,' so we often accept, uncritically, what's on offer. We take drugs without really knowing what effects they should have, their expected results and timescale, or their review period, because they may not help us as they have others. Many participants in pain clinics tell us that they didn't ask about what the impact (or side effects) of their treatment might be. Many treatments are only partly effective; when pain continues after treatment, there are often limited options. And without knowing the detail of their condition, people hear about alternative or new treatments but have no way of knowing whether each is of value for them. Chronic pain continues.

People with chronic pain can inhabit a world of uncertainty, anxiety and often isolation. In turn, this can create a depressing downward cycle into hopelessness, particularly if they don't have a good relationship with their doctor. When people are isolated or depressed, there is another important consequence to their pain – it changes how they think. They become more negative perhaps, can't see opportunities, stop using new information well, or stop laughing or appreciating the humour and absurdity in their situation. Anything new can become a cause for more anxiety and deeper depression.

You may have had contact with well-meaning folk who, unwittingly, tell you to 'try to stay positive' when things are bad. Or those who say they are concerned but whose eyes glaze over the moment you try to explain how you really feel. Even worse are those who appear to be encouraging but whose questions ('Why did you wait this long for surgery?') imply that, somehow, your problems are of your own making. Sometimes being with 'sympathetic people' ends up making you feel worse than ever! Living with pain can be unbelievably wearing and disheartening. Anxiety and depression make things worse. At best, pain is annoying and inconvenient. But it can also be frightening and severely limiting. Powerful drugs and pain management techniques are all around. But they don't necessarily work for everyone, every minute. And the more you use some of them, the less effective they become.

So, for the last 60 years, clinicians and researchers who specialise in treating pain have been rethinking what can be done.

One key step forward has been evidence that the old view – that pain levels are determined by the extent of your injury or disease – is wrong. We now understand the mechanics through which psychological factors have a significant effect on the body. People differ, and two individuals with the same condition may experience pain very differently. We know blanket drug treatments for pain don't work for people with chronic pain. Pain science now emphasises personalised solutions. Knowing how your brain and nerves work together, the importance of your perspective, how you react and the pain control tools that work for you will reduce your pain and limit the impact it has.

REMEMBER THIS!!! Reading this book will help us to learn *what our pain really is* and *how to become a pain manager ourselves.*

A Personal, Self-managed Pain Improvement Plan

Telling people with chronic pain to 'take control of your situation, manage the pain and learn to cope better' always prompts the question 'How?' It can also provoke frustration and appear glib if the person giving advice hasn't suffered themselves. Some people feel criticised and take personal offence, such as the person who told me about their recent visit to hospital: 'I have enough problems – I need help, not to be told I'm being weak if I don't do something about it myself.'

This reaction may be understandable, but we need to move past it in order to understand how you can manage pain effectively through self-management. Almost certainly you are coping with your pain 'as best you can', but modern pain management might improve your 'best'. It involves systematically looking at how you experience pain and recognising the situations, times and contexts when it is worst – knowing what causes the pain and what risks making it worse. It involves learning about the dominant role of the brain and central nervous system, their effect on how you feel and how to change those effects.

To manage chronic pain, you need to:

- Understand yourself and how you really deal with your pain. First, know yourself, take responsibility for your own condition and don't allow others (not even your doctors and nurses) to take over.
- Treat self-managing pain as a job, collecting information about what you experience, learning about why it happens, exploring what solutions have worked for others and trying them out for yourself, and discussing your conclusions with others.
- Make sure you spend time doing things which make you feel good, rather than just dealing with problems or the less good aspects of life; manage any tendency to think negatively; keep the things which make you feel happy and secure always in your mind and value them.
- Plan and organise your life, taking account of the inevitable recovery time you need but making room for activity to build the potential for your recovery.
- Know what tools, aids, techniques or equipment can make life easier.
- Then, make a basic, personalised pain management plan to start taking back control of the pain and boosting your resilience. Remember to 'keep it simple'. You can develop it later, as you make progress.

REMEMBER THIS!!! Creating a plan is a vital first step to making pain control a reality. But don't rush into creating your personal plan until you've got to grips with the ideas presented in Part One.

The start of your pain management planning must involve gaining more knowledge – understanding how the pain is triggered, its effects on you, what your nervous systems are doing and how to get your immune system to produce a calming effect. But managing pain and the underlying illness causing it requires more than just knowledge. You will need also to learn to *do* things differently, from special breathing and movements, to pain minimisation techniques, planning your day, controlling your emotions, avoiding automatic pilot thinking, using pain-friendly tools, and much more. There are four main steps to building the plan:

- **First**, review your situation. Use a notebook or diary to record your pain and its effects; factors which are likely to affect the severity and impact; your general well-being and sources of help. The questionnaires on the next few pages will help you get started.
- **Second**, read **Part One** of the book to inform yourself about how pain mechanisms work and how your perceptions and thoughts affect them.

- **Third**, read **Part Two**, which highlights factors that pain patients say affect their ability to self-manage pain. If you make a note of things you need to work on, ideas you would like to explore and what the questionnaires may tell you about yourself, you will have the raw material for your plan.
- **Fourth**, increase your options about what self-managing pain can mean for you. For example, keeping a pain diary and using the Pain Management Wheel will help you to craft your pain management plan.
- Finally, discuss your ideas with friends, other patients and your medical team, to be sure what you can do yourself safely, and how they can help you to monitor progress.

Assessing Your Own Pain

A review of your situation is the first step towards taking control. Here are two short questionnaires that ask you about your life and the pain you have. Used extensively in pain clinics, they are often very helpful – so take sufficient time to complete them carefully. No scoring is involved with the first one – its purpose is to encourage you to think things through and make notes for a discussion with your doctor or medical adviser. There is a scoresheet for the second questionnaire, which you should complete before moving on to Part One of the book.

QUESTIONNAIRES

Before you begin, recognise that people often complete questionnaires in ways that describe what they want others to think – instead of how they really feel. That will do you no favours here – be honest with yourself. Also, because others can see things we don't, you might want to check your answers with someone you trust.

Questionnaire 1:
Assess Your Pain

There is no pass or fail score with this questionnaire, because it was designed to record how you feel at this stage and provide information for discussion with your doctor. Conversations with your medical adviser will be more useful if you can discuss specific, tangible information about what has happened to you.

Write your responses to this questionnaire and other activities from the book in a notebook specifically for pain management. We'll look more at how you can use it towards the end of Part Two.

Mark your responses to each question, using the scales below:

How bothersome has your pain been in the last few days?

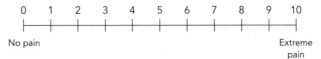

How intense is your pain now?

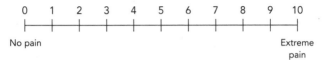

How intense was your pain, on average, last week?

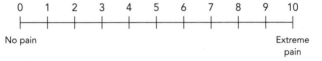

* * *

Now please use the same method to describe some effects of the pain.

How distressing is your pain to you now?

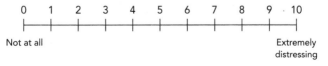

How distressed has it made you, on average, over the last month?

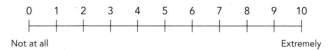

0 1 2 3 4 5 6 7 8 9 10

Not at all   Extremely

To what extent does your pain interfere with your normal daily life?

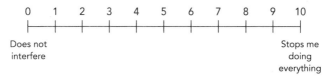

0 1 2 3 4 5 6 7 8 9 10

Does not interfere   Stops me doing everything

* * *

To what extent do you agree or disagree with the following statements?

In the last few days, I have dressed more slowly than usual because of my pain.

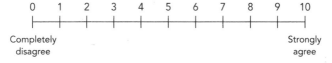

0 1 2 3 4 5 6 7 8 9 10

Completely disagree   Strongly agree

In the last few days, I have only walked short distances because of my pain.

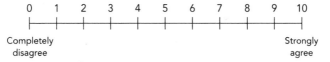

0 1 2 3 4 5 6 7 8 9 10

Completely disagree   Strongly agree

It's really not safe for a person with a condition like mine to be physically active.

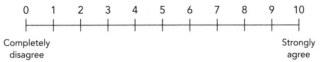

| 0 | 1 | 2 | 3 | 4 | 5 | 6 | 7 | 8 | 9 | 10 |

Completely disagree — Strongly agree

Worrying thoughts have been going through my mind a lot of the time in the last few days.

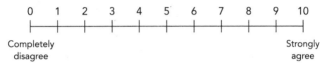

| 0 | 1 | 2 | 3 | 4 | 5 | 6 | 7 | 8 | 9 | 10 |

Completely disagree — Strongly agree

I feel that my pain is terrible and that it is never going to get any better.

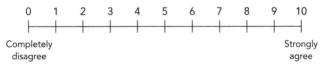

| 0 | 1 | 2 | 3 | 4 | 5 | 6 | 7 | 8 | 9 | 10 |

Completely disagree — Strongly agree

In general, in the last few days, I have not enjoyed all the things I used to enjoy.

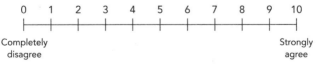

| 0 | 1 | 2 | 3 | 4 | 5 | 6 | 7 | 8 | 9 | 10 |

Completely disagree — Strongly agree

* * *

If you have had any treatment for your pain, how much has this taken away the pain?

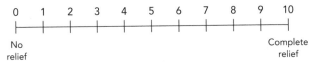

```
0    1    2    3    4    5    6    7    8    9    10
```
No   Complete
relief   relief

If you have someone with you who knows how to help deal with your pain, how well organised are they?
(If you don't have anyone with you who helps, skip this and go to next question.)

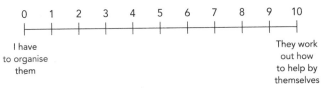

```
0    1    2    3    4    5    6    7    8    9    10
```
I have   They work
to organise   out how
them   to help by
                                          themselves

To what extent do people you see really help with your pain?

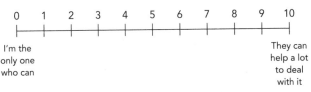

```
0    1    2    3    4    5    6    7    8    9    10
```
I'm the   They can
only one   help a lot
who can   to deal
                                            with it

How much do you find yourself thinking about your pain?

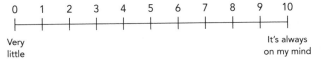

```
0    1    2    3    4    5    6    7    8    9    10
```
Very   It's always
little   on my mind

When you try to do other things, how does it feel?

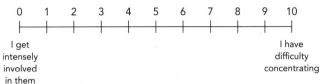

```
0    1    2    3    4    5    6    7    8    9    10
├────┼────┼────┼────┼────┼────┼────┼────┼────┼────┤
```
I get   I have
intensely   difficulty
involved   concentrating
in them

Overall, pain aside, how do you feel things have been going in your life?

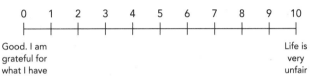

```
0    1    2    3    4    5    6    7    8    9    10
├────┼────┼────┼────┼────┼────┼────┼────┼────┼────┤
```
Good. I am   Life is
grateful for   very
what I have   unfair

How frequently do you feel stressed?

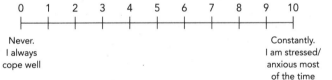

```
0    1    2    3    4    5    6    7    8    9    10
├────┼────┼────┼────┼────┼────┼────┼────┼────┼────┤
```
Never.   Constantly.
I always   I am stressed/
cope well   anxious most
                                         of the time

Do you have any idea what a C fibre does?
(If not, don't worry, we'll discuss them later.)

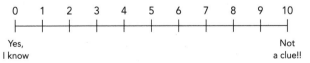

```
0    1    2    3    4    5    6    7    8    9    10
├────┼────┼────┼────┼────┼────┼────┼────┼────┼────┤
```
Yes,   Not
I know   a clue!!

Questionnaire 2:
The Effects of Chronic Pain

This second questionnaire concerns the effects of pain and difficulties you have coping with the condition that causes it. It will help you to think about your plan of action and ask what is really best for you. Information about scoring the questionnaire is given afterwards.

For each of the statements below, circle the number which most closely reflects how you have been feeling in the past week. Ignore which column (A or B) the numbers are in. Don't take too long over your replies: your instinctive answer is best. You will be able to score and interpret your answers using the scoring sheet on page 27.

A	B	
		I feel tense or 'wound up':
	3	Most of the time
	2	A lot of the time
	1	From time to time
	0	Not at all
		I still enjoy the things I used to enjoy:
0		Definitely as much
1		Not quite so much
2		Only a little
3		Hardly at all

A	B	
		I get a sort of frightened feeling as if something awful is about to happen:
	3	Very definitely and quite badly
	2	Yes, but not too badly
	1	A little, but it doesn't worry me
	0	Not at all
		I can laugh and see the funny side of things:
0		As much as I always could
1		Not quite so much now
2		Definitely not so much now
3		Not at all
		Worrying thoughts go through my mind:
	3	Most of the time
	2	A lot of the time
	1	From time to time, but not too often
	0	Hardly ever
		I feel cheerful:
3		Not at all
2		Not often
1		Sometimes
0		Most of the time

A	B	
		I can sit at ease and feel relaxed:
	0	Very often
	1	Usually
	2	Not often
	3	Not at all
		I feel as if I am slowed down:
3		Nearly all the time
2		Very often
1		Sometimes
0		Not at all
		I get a sort of frightened feeling like 'butterflies' in the stomach:
	0	Not at all
	1	Occasionally
	2	Quite often
	3	Very often
		I have lost interest in my appearance:
3		Definitely
2		I don't take as much care as I did
1		I may take just a bit less care
0		I take just as much care as ever

A	B	
		I feel restless as I have to be on the move:
	3	Very much
	2	Quite a lot
	1	Not very much
	0	Not at all
		I look forward with enjoyment to things:
0		As much as I ever did
1		Rather less than I used to
2		Much less than I used to
3		Hardly at all
		I get sudden feelings of panic:
	3	Very often
	2	Quite often
	1	Not very often
	0	Not at all
		I can enjoy a good book or radio or TV programme:
0		Most of the time
1		Sometimes
2		Not often
3		Very seldom

Scoring Sheet for Questionnaire 2

Please add up all the numbers you have circled for column A and put the total below. Then do the same for all the numbers you circled in column B.

Total score: Column A _____   Column B _____

Interpretation

This questionnaire was concerned with your resilience and the well-being needed to take control of your situation. The two columns are designed to help you, your family and doctor to understand how you are feeling, and to help you to think about how to start managing your pain. The principle here is that pain experienced over a long period begins to affect how you think, how positive you are and your ability to make the best of your situation.

Column A gives you a score for depression, which is about low mood and a sense of hopelessness which can be overwhelming. Column B gives you a score for anxiety. Taken together, the scores are a good measure of the psychological distress pain can cause – including a generally low mood, a tendency towards negativity (anticipating the worst outcomes) and a decline in your resilience or ability to keep going. The intention of this book is to help you find ways of making life better despite your pain. High scores for depression and anxiety will get in the way of that.

If you scored **between 0 and 7** on either column, you are probably coping pretty well and managing to see the positives around you. Read the book at your leisure and, when it feels appropriate, talk to your doctor about your plan and what you are considering trying out.

A score **between 8 and 10** on either column is 'borderline'. It suggests that the situation is beginning to take its toll on you. Consider setting yourself a deadline for reading this book, thinking about your condition and seeing your medical adviser to work out a plan before the pain makes you feel any worse.

A score of **11 or above** (particularly if you get high scores for both columns) indicates that your pain may be having a significant effect on you, and it would be reasonable to assume that you could struggle to take self-management on just now. While there are always problems with questionnaires and they can never be 100 per cent accurate, you might think of having a chat with your doctor soon, to discuss the anxieties you feel and any problems you foresee playing a larger part in managing your own pain.

PART ONE
Understanding Chronic Pain

Chapters 2–4 are designed to increase your knowledge of nociception (pain processes in your body) and to clarify how nerves, emotions and thinking styles play a vital role in the pain you experience. If you really want to take control of your pain, spend as much time as you need on these chapters, until you feel familiar and comfortable with the ideas they describe. Then you can move on to Chapter 5, to look at what's involved with self-managing pain.

---

2. What Is Pain for?

For most people, pain is an unpleasant experience to be avoided. It can provoke real discomfort and anxiety, especially when we are unsure about what causes it. This isn't surprising because one of the main functions of pain is to let us know that something is wrong – our physical well-being is in danger and we need to change what we are doing to deal with it.

The pain sensation is part of a system controlled by our brains called nociception. This system processes information from our bodies about potential risk. The brain may conclude that we are at risk of tissue damage, for example, if there is a harmful cause or stimulus (like a hot surface) we must avoid. This system creates reactions in many parts of our bodies by using our nervous and hormonal systems: by increasing blood pressure, changing heart rate, sending blood to inflame areas of tissues, triggering emotional reactions and perhaps instantly getting our muscles to withdraw from the harmful stimulus. A summary of this and relevant research is explained in more detail in Chapter 3.

Types of Pain

We could experience pain following an injury, such as a fracture or bruise. Pain from other causes (like cancer, arthritis or diabetes) is just as real but the immediate cause can be less obvious. Acute pain is sharp and distressing, but usually goes away when treated and the injury begins to heal. Opioid medicines (heavy-duty painkillers) may be needed for severe acute pain, but usually only for a short time. The dose of opioid should be reduced as healing progresses.

 Acute pain is an alarm signal that something is happening which you need to do something about. Most minor pains get better on their own or with simple treatment, but more severe pain may be a sign of something serious, like a fracture, infection or underlying condition. Childbirth is a more positive example. Acute pain is helpful because it makes you get treatment and rest until the cause has been resolved or the condition relieved.

Chronic pain can have a huge impact on daily life, restricting activity, with anxiety and psychological distress compounding physical problems. This type of pain can result from serious underlying problems, but it is most frequently experienced when a non-threatening condition cannot be easily or quickly cured. Unlike acute pain, it can continue despite getting treatment. It is difficult to cope with, but appears to serve no useful purpose.

Opioids are often used as medicines because they contain chemicals that relax the body and can relieve pain. Prescription opioids are used mostly to treat moderate to severe pain, although some opioids can be used to treat more minor conditions, such as coughing and diarrhoea.

Doctors give careful thought to prescribing medicines (and opioids in particular) especially if needed for pain. Often, the longer they are taken, the less effective they become. (See page 173.) Opioids can make people feel very relaxed and 'high' – which is why they are sometimes used recreationally by people who don't need them for pain relief. There is a strong probability of addiction from using heavy-duty painkillers for long periods, and this is seen as a huge problem in countries like the USA, Canada and Australia, and in Western Europe.

Chronic, or **long-term**, **pain** can be caused by conditions such as back problems, osteoarthritis or rheumatoid arthritis, fibromyalgia, nerve problems, surgical issues, sleeplessness or migraines. Causes of the pain may be less clear if someone has multiple health concerns, and social and psychological effects can become more significant as time goes on. Pain can continue for months or years, and the effects of treatment may be gradual rather than immediate.

Pain that comes and goes, like a headache, is called 'recurrent' pain and is often a characteristic of long-term conditions. Osteoarthritis, for example, can be much less of a problem after the morning's initial 'getting going' stiffness has abated. However, chronic pain can become intolerable because pain hurts. It can cause low mood, irritability, poor sleep and may reduce the ability to participate or get around. Unlike acute pain, chronic pain is difficult to treat, with some estimates suggesting that less than a third of pain patients feel their treatment to have been of real impact.

THINK ABOUT IT

Despite medication, studies of patients with chronic fibromyalgia and rheumatoid and osteo-arthritis have found that most patients' pain levels increase on cold, overcast or wet days following high barometric pressure. Despite individuals' sensitivity to weather conditions varying, pain levels also increase with changes in humidity from one day to the next. As you read the sections of the book on how the brain interacts with our nervous systems, you might want to reflect on how the brain interprets temperature or humidity information.

An important issue for self-managing chronic pain is that the same treatments may not work for people with the same or similar pain-producing conditions. For some people, medication has been *less* effective than other treatments, such as electrical stimulation techniques, acupuncture, physical exercise programmes and physiotherapy; or psychological treatments such as cognitive behavioural therapy (CBT), mindfulness or meditation techniques – visualisation, yoga or breathing awareness.

Neuropathic pain (NeP) relates to a type of pain associated with injury to nerves or the nervous systems. Types of NeP include sciatica following disc prolapse, nerve injury following spinal surgery, infection such as shingles or HIV/Aids, diabetes, pain after amputation (phantom limb or stump pain) and pain associated with multiple sclerosis or strokes.

Inflammatory pain occurs when chemicals (prostaglandins) and proteins (some cytokines) from white blood cells are released into the bloodstream or affected tissues to protect the body. This release of chemicals increases the blood flow to the area of injury or infection and may result in redness and heat. Some of the chemicals cause a leak of fluid into the tissues, resulting in swelling. This protective process can stimulate nerves, triggering a painful reaction. In some diseases, like rheumatoid arthritis, the body's defence system – the immune system – triggers an inflammatory response when there are no foreign invaders to fight off. In these diseases, called autoimmune diseases, the body's normally protective immune system causes damage to its own tissues. The body responds as if normal tissues were infected or somehow abnormal.

What's your own experience of different types of pain? In your notebook, record your answers to the following:

- Have you experienced pain which lasted six months or more? Do you know what caused it? Which parts of your body were affected?

- What effect did your pain have on you and have the effects continued?

Why Does Pain Feel So Bad?

Imagine you were to stub your toe, bang your elbow, or sustain a more severe injury. I'm sure you can imagine how the pain would feel. It's a very unpleasant sensation, but a subjective one because two people may have different pain 'thresholds' or 'tolerances'.

The terms 'pain threshold' and 'pain tolerance' are commonly used interchangeably but, really, they refer to different things. **Pain threshold** is when we *first feel a stimulus as being painful*. Holding your hand towards a fire feels good at first, then hot, then painful. **Pain tolerance**, by contrast, defines *how long a person can take the pain before breaking down* or how intense the pain needs to be before it is intolerable. Both vary from person to person. Pain patients may have a lower threshold because they know what the signs are and process pain feelings quickly, but they may have a higher tolerance because they are used to living with it and have adapted to it.

Acute pains following injury or serious health concerns tend to be sharp, immediate sensations which are highly localised and accompanied by automatic reactions (such as sweating, and increased heart, breathing and respiration rates). They may be combined with chronic pain symptoms, which tend to feel more continuous: aching, perhaps, or throbbing. Chronic symptoms can be continuous, invasive, disabling. While they can be caused by serious problems like injuries not healing properly, nerve damage, orthopaedic damage, cancer and the like, they may also be caused by conditions like arthritis, migraines, fibromyalgia or back pain – unpleasant, but not life-threatening. These conditions might not have a reliable cure and, if not, the pain is sometimes thought of as something we may just need to learn to live with.

Managing your condition is more difficult if you haven't understood what you have been told about it or the treatment you have been offered. You may have been told you are suffering from some form of general condition but with a specific label. For example, arthritis could be more specifically labelled 'ankylosing spondylitis'. To fully understand what you're dealing with, what causes pain or makes it worse and what to expect from the treatment, it's likely you will really need to get to grips with jargon. Good clinicians help by explaining the technical language, but don't be afraid to ask questions until you understand clearly.

Pain Can Be Strange and Counter-intuitive

In 1664, French philosopher René Descartes imagined pain in the way many still do today. He thought that pain was a simple signal to the brain about an injury, and that the level of pain told you how bad the damage was. Today we know that the brain plays a central role but that pain is not a one-way signal. We also know that the level of pain is not linked to the severity of the damage.

Descartes also described a condition known as phantom limb pain, in which real pain exists in a place where a lost or amputated limb used to be. Today, this pain is frequently experienced by soldiers as well as patients who have had serious accidents.

With no limb to trigger it, the pain can't be explained by the simple view of pain as a signalling system. In response, Descartes offered another sophisticated thought: 'Even if part of the body is cut off, nothing has thereby been taken away from the mind.' Despite a simplistic idea of pain signalling, his major contribution to the field was clarifying that our physical senses are unreliable and that the mind and body are fundamentally connected.

So, pain is much more complicated and interesting than it may appear. Here are a few examples from recent research that show just how counter-intuitive pain can be:

- An unusual clinical study of people who perceived themselves as being *in love*, found that *thinking about their partners relieved around half their pain*.[1]
- Studies showed that simply *looking at a painful hand* or arm through a magnifying glass *made it subsequently more swollen and painful* when moved.[2]

- Research demonstrated that *getting an injection really does hurt less when you don't watch the needle going in*.[3]
- An important study showed that, following injury, people who were fearful of pain and *catastrophised* (see page 66) experienced increased and prolonged pain compared to those who didn't catastrophise.[4]
- Another study found that *children's real pain level is strongly influenced by things they've seen and heard* – past problems, how their parents react to pain themselves, how they have been told to react – and the distress their parents show.[5]

Some years ago, I worked with soldiers experiencing post-traumatic stress (PTSD). I decided to read up on some aspects of military psychiatry, finding examples from both the Second World War and the Korean War that showed the complexity of how pain occurs. Despite being seriously injured, in the heat of battle soldiers would continue to fight with little awareness of pain. The distraction of battle and focus on survival allowed the brain to eclipse the sensations involved. The context altered their perception of what they were experiencing. When soldiers with combat fatigue were placed with physically sick or wounded individuals they began, unconsciously, to experience the same feelings and physical limitations as the other patients. In other cases, soldiers with serious or life-threatening injuries being rehabilitated away from the front frequently refused medication; subsequently, researchers have established that pain is less painful when we are confident that we are safe.

The predominant view reflecting current research is that the level of pain you feel is determined in the brain, not by damaged tissues. The evidence for this viewpoint has been collected from many sources. Examples include:

- People with hip pain suffer more when their doctors don't describe it as 'normal age-related changes' but instead use words like 'degeneration of the bone'.
- If you are a dancer and injure your toes, it will hurt more than if you were an artist or shopkeeper. The dancer perceives more danger and risk to their life and livelihood.
- If someone puts an ice cube on your hand illuminated by a red light, it will be more painful than if it were illuminated by a blue light.
- People with chronic pain find that they no longer feel it when they have a new, acute pain to cope with.
- Practitioners of mindfulness are seemingly able to tolerate greater levels of pain than other people.
- Parental beliefs and words alone can increase or reduce the amount of pain their children experience.
- Visualising ideas (like gates opening and closing) or gently touching and stroking a pain site can effectively reduce pain and discomfort.

Since the Second World War, researchers have been trying to understand just how the pain response works, both physically and psychologically. Although many questions remain to be answered, we have developed more advanced research methods over the years and built a much clearer understanding about the mechanisms involved. (We will explore this more fully in Chapter 3.) The brain critically evaluates every danger message it receives – considering it in the context of everything else the brain is aware of, then deciding how important it is, and what level of pain should enter our consciousness.

So, each message must answer a very important question: 'How dangerous is what's happened?' The answer will be determined by drawing on every piece of credible information the brain has: previous injuries, cultural influences, emotions, and other sensory cues. But as if the brain's decision weren't complicated enough, it seeks even more data. Extensive recent evidence suggests that when we are at risk, the brain instructs the nervous systems to be more sensitive to *any possibility of things getting worse*. It does so by changing the structure and chemical composition of peripheral nerves to register as a possible threat even sensations that have no connection with the original pain stimulus, such as anxiety or uncertainty. Researchers have observed this process by measuring increased pain in patients sitting in medical waiting rooms with explicit pictures of medical procedures on the wall.

Our pain systems have evolved to make us do something about our injuries, any damage we've incurred or the dangers we are in. Our perceptions, outlook and thoughts have a major impact on the pain we feel. The sensation we get feels real, but pain is subjective, susceptible to its circumstances. It is not unchangeable.

CASE STUDY

Elliott, aged 62, was an engineer who had back pain and fibromyalgia which caused fatigue, widespread pain and tenderness throughout his body. Unable to work for two years, he was hooked on strong painkillers, usually taking more pills than the recommended dose. My first contact, encouraging him to see the importance of learning about his pain, was not positive. Elliott thought that attending the pain clinic was an example of his doctor's belief that he was pretending, or that the doctor had no other treatments to offer. He was looking for medical experts to give him solutions, not to 'get into his mind'.

He was very cautious but agreed to meet with other chronic pain sufferers on a weekly basis to explore how pain is created in the body and the way his outlook is an important part of it. Tending to make dismissive comments, he annoyed others in the group, particularly by asserting that they were in a hopeless situation with little prospect of improvement.

However, although outwardly resistant, Elliott had been listening. At home, he had tried out some of the techniques recommended for him, with positive results. He showed real courage three weeks later when he apologised to everyone in the group about his behaviour and began to participate positively.

A year after completing the clinic sessions he proudly told me: 'Despite the back pain and fibromyalgia, I am in control of it now and I am really enjoying life again. Because I can relax more and understand how tension affects me, I know which part of my body isn't at ease and I know maybe I haven't prepared properly, or planned when/how to do things. And I can do something about it. I try to swim every day, but sometimes I just need to do a breathing or mindfulness exercise … or give myself permission to take it easy and stop trying so hard. I have regular reviews with my doctor – not about fibromyalgia really – it's about how's the plan going and who can help. I haven't taken any painkillers – of any kind – for the whole of last year. I think that I was at war – but with myself.'

Elliott's experience shows that understanding how his own pain works and building a plan from that (which in his case controlled his emotions and stress) has been as valuable as a plan focused on exercise and medication. Sticking with it has had a real, physical effect in his body, and he doesn't need painkillers any more.

3. Important Ideas about Pain

In 1977, New York psychiatrist George Engel compiled a general model of pain and healing which has come to be known as the '**bio-psycho-social framework**'. Engel suggested that there are three categories of factor involved in producing your pain. The workings of your body, your mind and your social setting each have a part to play, varying from person to person. 'As a result,' he said, 'for any particular condition, pain levels and coping strategies will vary from one person to another.' The influence of the mind on physical health had been discussed since the 1930s, but Engel's contribution about the importance of social relationships and the individual nature of pain was new.

It was a simple idea, grounded in his work with patients, but not one which gained much traction at the time among some people (both doctors and people suffering chronic pain) who saw medical science in very traditional terms. For them – and for many contemporary traditionalists – science had to use evidence to prove ideas which could then be applicable to everyone. Any suggestion of psychological links seemed too vague or intangible. This is particularly difficult for people who have been trained to think scientifically, doubting ideas until hard evidence about the way things work mechanically can be produced.

It took nearly 35 years after Engel's work for clinicians and neurologists to amass a sufficiently large body of evidence about pain to convince a sceptical scientific audience that the brain can not only change perceptions of pain, but can also explain the physical mechanisms by which pain is created, and the way relationships and feelings of security affect the physical functioning of our nervous systems.

Many people with pain themselves are resistant to the idea that our emotions and thoughts can directly affect our health – imagining instead that the mind operates as a separate entity, immune to the anxiety, pains and strain we feel. Saying that the effects of illness (pain and physical disability) are 'all in your mind', 'psychosomatic' or 'psychological' is seen by most people as a damning accusation – a suggestion that you are exaggerating or imagining the effects, or that you are making it up.

When some sceptical clinicians told ill people that their chronic fatigue (ME), Gulf War Syndrome or repetitive strain pain was 'all in the mind', they did untold damage. There is a world of difference between being told something is 'all in your mind' and acknowledging that emotions and attitudes can influence your state of health or capacity to cope, for better or worse. For those of us with chronic pain, looking at how the mind–body connection affects us personally is a hugely valuable step towards managing pain better and learning to live with it. For anyone seeking more evidence or examples about this key issue, there are some thought-provoking examples at the end of this chapter.

So, we have learned a great deal about chronic pain over the last 42 years. We will explore current thinking about the mechanisms which create it in the next section. A key advance has been this recognition that the mind–body connection is a major driver for chronic pain: emotions and thoughts can create depressive thinking patterns and reduce your resilience, but they can also trigger physical changes to brain structures, chemistry and the functioning of our nervous systems.

Brain structures like the amygdala and hippocampus, which affect memory, thinking and emotional control, can become 10–15 per cent smaller in people who have suffered chronic pain for more than a year.

Chronic pain also causes increasing shrinkage of the sheathing of nerves (myelin). Critically, this affects nerve fibres in the central nervous system (brain and spinal cord), and recovery can be a very slow process. Damage activates inflammatory responses in the central nervous system, sensitising peripheral nerve pathways and, in turn, lowering pain thresholds. A very important advance has been our understanding that many people's chronic pain is a consequence of an over-sensitised nervous system.

Neuroscience researchers found a perhaps even more important consequence of highly sensitised nervous systems: pain can result from sensitised cells not switching off – continuing to send information perceived as pain even when any threat or risk of damage has gone. Over-sensitised nerve cells can produce a constant awareness of pain which does not always reflect the current seriousness of the condition or injury.

 One thing seems certain from research into pain: there is no single 'pain centre' in the brain, whose activity alone could account for the many ways in which the brain deals with pain-related information. *There is no one part of the brain that could be surgically removed to eliminate all pain.* Pain is a complex phenomenon with many physical, nerve, emotional and thinking (cognitive) dimensions.

Pain Mechanisms

We have seen that chronic pain is complex, but now let's look at the mechanisms that create pain in more detail. For example, what happens when you stub your toe on a rock?

At first, pain-sensitive (nociceptive) fibres in your toe send impulses to your spinal cord, relaying them through your nervous systems to your brain. As we have seen, the brain is seeking anything unusual, amplifying any potential symptoms to make you more aware of potential risk. Neural networks (involving the hippocampus and amygdala) use the information the brain receives to make you aware of the problem. If necessary, the pain makes you jump. The neural networks instantly instruct your muscles to jump back from the rock (and rub your toe vigorously).

But that's not the end of it. Chemical messengers (neurotransmitters) are then used to increase the sensitivity of the nerves around the injury in case there are any further signs of risk or damage which require a response. The pain you feel can be intense, regardless of the actual injury, and the nerves can remain highly sensitive for hours and days afterwards. The mechanisms within our pain network (the brain, neurotransmitters, central nervous system, peripheral nervous system and nociceptive fibres) are designed to be highly sensitive to risk rather than measuring injury. Anything the brain unconsciously reads as a threat prompts it to look for more information from the nerves, so-called 'top-down regulation', using glial cells in the central nervous system to manage the process.

So, following the initial nerve signals from your toe, the brain uses glial cells in the central nervous system, in effect to instruct the peripheral nerves to be more sensitive to anything going on – just in case! The downside of this is that nerves throughout the body can become hyper-sensitive to any problem – even relatively unimportant ones. Acting in the same way as before, they send alarm signals back up to the brain to be processed in the context of what else has been happening. Previous pain episodes, fear, anxiety, predictions of pain, other problems you may have to cope with, previous psychological conditioning about how to react – all of these come into play even when the nerves have picked up something which might be unimportant, such as a twinge or stiffness or an ache which just needs time to go away.

When people see you are in pain, they see the effects created by your brain. What they can't see, of course, is that despite your ache not being life-threatening, your nervous systems are still on full alert, using anything which might be a problem to alarm you, by creating pain.

The case study which follows is about Descartes' 'phantom limb' phenomenon, which we discussed earlier. But beyond the particulars of this phenomenon, the example describes the role of the brain – how it perceives and understands problems – in reducing an individual's experience of real pain.

Vilayanur S. Ramachandran is a neurologist and pain scientist who, in 1998, provoked a great deal of debate in general medicine when he argued that pain is the brain's 'opinion on your position and state of health, rather than a mere reflective response to an injury'.

Ramachandran tells the extraordinary story of a man cured of phantom limb pain that had tortured him with spasms in a clenched fist that was no longer there.

With a clever arrangement of mirrors, Ramachandran created the illusion that the man's amputated arm had been restored – a 'virtual' limb – using the reflection of his other, uninjured arm. The mere *appearance* of his phantom hand opening and closing normally for a few minutes cured his agonising pain.

His brain's 'opinion on his state of health' had changed. The illusion of recovery allowed his brain to recognise that apparent pain signals were phantoms. So, there was no need for the pain.

The direction of pain research was fundamentally altered in the 1960s when Ronald Melzack and Patrick Wall looked at nerve and brain functions involved in pain control to understand just how the brain registers and controls what is perceived as pain. They explored the way nerves are involved and how signals are communicated to the brain. Nerve impulses relating to severe risk (producing acute pain) are transmitted up from the body through thick, insulated or myelinated ('A') fibres to the brain. Impulses relating to injury that involves lower risk (usually producing chronic pain) are conducted by thin, uninsulated ('C') fibres. As described above, it is believed that the absence of insulation (myelin) around C fibres explains why chronic pain can be felt in a variety of locations in the body, not just in one localised area of damage.

How Quickly Does the Brain Register Pain?

	Nerve Type	Speed meters/second
Body Awareness, Temperature, Balance	A-alpha	80–120 Jet aircraft
Touch	A-beta	35–90 Racing car
Temperature Change, Inflammation, Acute Pain	A-delta	4–40 Racing bike
Longer-term or Chronic Pain	C	0.5–2 Walking pace

The difference between the speeds at which the A and C nerve fibres conduct information to the brain explains why, when you damage your toe, you feel a sharp, specific pain first, then moments later a more diffuse, dull ache or pain. Your pain from long-term chronic conditions results from information carried through the C nerve fibres more slowly than the acute pain through A fibres.

THINK ABOUT IT It is important to recognise that there are no 'pain nerves'. *Nerves do not detect pain.* They only detect disturbances of some kind in your body – stimuli. Your brain decides then whether you should feel pain, how severely and how to react. That decision is influenced by a variety of factors, explained in the next chapter.

A Neuroscience Revolution

In the early 1990s, novel brain-imaging techniques and immunology advances opened up a formerly undreamed-of capacity to understand how the brain processes information and its connections with our nervous systems. The brain is a complicated set of regions that link together to create awareness, evaluate risks and decide how the body should react. The regions which do that are connected by nerve fibres, and when they regularly need to connect (which happens with chronic conditions), a 'neural pathway' is formed.

Pain alters the way some areas of the brain respond, building new pathways which can spread or amplify the pain's effect. Neuroscientists call this set of neural pathways the '**pain matrix**', and PET scans (positron emission tomography) and fMRI scans (functional magnetic resonance imaging) have enabled us to see this activity at work in different parts of the brain.

One part of the brain (the **reticular formation**) receives information and triggers awareness and alertness associated with pain. It sends messages that change heart rate, arterial blood pressure, respiration, and other vital functions associated with pain. It is also the reticular formation that allows a pain stimulus to go unnoticed if your attention is diverted, like being focused on an interesting or important task.

Signals from the nervous systems alert the **hypothalamus** to any factors that suggest the body is not regulating itself properly. It responds by releasing hormones into the

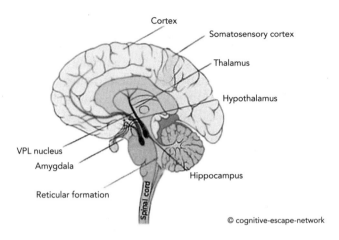

Cortex
Somatosensory cortex
Thalamus
Hypothalamus
VPL nucleus
Amygdala
Hippocampus
Reticular formation
Spinal cord

© cognitive-escape-network

Pain-related structures in the brain

bloodstream to keep the body in balance – for example, triggering inflammation to protect injuries or influencing temperature, perspiration and emotions to boost awareness of the problem.

The **thalamus** is a brain structure that acts like a giant switchbox for sensory signals. There, the nerve impulses link to other structures (**VPL nucleus** and **somatosensory cortex**) to determine where and how much pain should be triggered. The **amygdala** (the emotional centre of the brain) and **hippocampus** (which plays an essential role in modifying memories about experiences) manage the risk of further damage through the 'top-down regulation' described in the previous section. The nerves in the central and peripheral nervous systems are primed to become more sensitive and to collect data about the risk of further damage, which in turn will be passed along the nerves in the spinal column.

So, chronic pain can be amplified by a highly sensitised nervous system registering every possible problem. There is strong neurological evidence that personal experiences, emotions and even norms and cultural heritage are activated when the pain matrix deals with information from the nervous systems.

In older people for example, chronic pain is often linked with depression, and may be a symptom of other conditions they have. If you are unable to get out and about normally, depression can develop into a serious problem. When this happens, pain often seems more severe and more widespread. Brain scans show that in people with depression and chronic pain, the prefrontal cortex, and temporal and parietal lobes (involved with thinking and problem solving), can be overwhelmed by activity in the limbic system, which governs emotions and relationships. Creating a downward spiral, depressive thinking offers little hope and creates a negative way of looking at events (even blocking awareness of anything positive), which is why many people describe chronic pain as 'suffering'. The pain is made worse by insecurity and anxiety, sometimes resulting in emotional, financial and relationship problems too.

The neuroscience 'revolution' has provided evidence that pain can become distanced from the basic function – changing our behaviour to protect ourselves. Instead, it often becomes part of a cycle of suffering. And, in such circumstances, rather than actively self-managing pain we may start to catastrophise, thinking, 'I am really ill and this is intolerable. I need to get better painkillers. Things will never get better. Nothing I try seems to work. I need doctors to give me better help.' It is the classic dependent patient role I talked about in the introduction and is a major problem for managing your pain better.

We've learned a lot in this chapter about how and why the brain creates pain. It's really important to understand and believe this before we try to take action. But, don't worry, in Part Two, we'll look at practical steps to change those brain processes and manage our pain, and we'll look at evidence from brain scans that some of the ideas described there have a tangible effect. For example, visualisation techniques affect the reticular formation, influencing perceptions of pain levels. Mindfulness modifies the function of the medial cortex and associated prefrontal cortex as well as the insula and amygdala, which reduces anxiety, increases physical calm, supports emotional balance, and increases capacity for thinking, problem solving and planning. Having a plan and collecting data engages the dominance of the frontal cortex over the emotional aspects of the limbic system, triggering the dopamine and reward (feel good) pathways from the nucleus accumbens. If the brain is crucial in the formation of chronic pain, we now know that it can help to modify and manage its effects too.

The brain can worry *too much*! From paper cuts to aching hips or fibromyalgia, it often overstates the danger. People who worry more experience more pain. Pain signals danger, and our brains can exaggerate that. To reduce chronic pain, we need to balance concerns about risk and physical damage with realism about the threat we face and awareness of our general well-being.

The following diagram recaps the process of nociception, that is, how the brain processes nerve impulses which result in pain. You can see that:

1 Immediately after detecting damage or significant risk, signals come from the peripheral nerves (PNS), through our central nervous system (CNS) to the brain, travelling at different speeds up the spinal column.

2 The brain then draws conclusions by involving the reticular formation, thalamus, amygdala, hippocampus, VPL nucleus and somatosensory cortex, and brings an initial pain sensation into our consciousness.

3 The brain then sends signals back through the central nervous system, using special (glial) cells to create inflammation and sensitise neurons in our peripheral nervous system. This tasks them with looking for any sensation which might cause a further problem.

4 In that event, the signals would again be sent to the brain via the central nervous system.

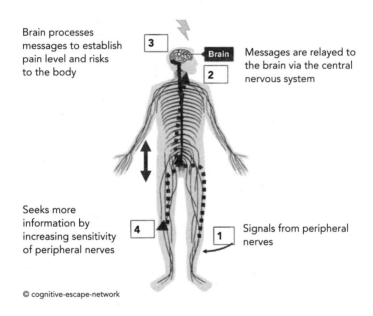

Brain processes messages to establish pain level and risks to the body

3

Brain

2

Messages are relayed to the brain via the central nervous system

Seeks more information by increasing sensitivity of peripheral nerves

4

1

Signals from peripheral nerves

© cognitive-escape-network

REMEMBER THIS!!!

- Your pain is not just related to the severity of the injury/condition triggering it.
- Many other factors influence your sense of threat (ranging from your own previous experience to

things on TV or you read in newspapers). These affect the way the brain reacts to nerve signals implying something is wrong.

- But, as if you needed reminding, *pain is real*. It's quite rare for it not to have a physical cause. I know from personal experience that pain hurts!
- There *are* things you can do to cope better with it.

Further Evidence for the Sceptics and the Undecided

Here are some more examples of the evidence for a tangible link between mind, outlook and physical health:

- In 1936, Hans Selye demonstrated connections between emotion and cells in the digestive system. It was the first understanding of irritable bowel syndrome (IBS).
- In 1974, cardiologists Friedman and Rosenman demonstrated how personality factors and life stress can trigger the distribution of catecholamines, epinephrine, nor-epinephrine and other hormones. These result, over time, in increased risk of cardiac disease.
- A 2001 study of the sisters of the Poor Clares order in Canada showed a clear link between pain and health problems and emotional well-being. Four hundred elderly nuns had written brief autobiographical sketches when they entered their convent, aged twenty. The sketches were analysed to identify how

positive or negative their individual perspectives were and how their attitudes and emotions differed. Since then, despite living comparable lives in very similar environments, those whose sketches contained few positive thoughts about their lives (and showed a more negative, risk-averse perspective) had required more medical treatments and died on average nine years sooner than those describing their early lives and situations positively.

- When, in 2002, researchers were exploring underlying reasons for pain-related drug and alcohol abuse and excessive smoking, they found similar physical changes to those found in people with depression. Over time, people who displayed negative thinking and emotions and anxiety developed changes in brain chemistry and neural connections. This led the American Society of Addiction Medicine (ASAM) to issue a new definition of addictive health, saying, 'At its core, addiction isn't just a health or social problem or a moral problem or a criminal problem. It's a *brain* problem whose behaviours manifest in all these other areas.'

- In 2003, neuroimaging studies demonstrated that the brain reacts to psychological injury in the same way as physical injury.

- In 2004, UK health guidelines (CSG4) recognised that cancer patients' quality of life and patients' ability to cope with pain were heavily influenced (positively and negatively) by their emotional response to the disease.

- In 1987, the *British Medical Journal* reported that a Southampton family doctor (K.B. Thomas) selected 200 patients who were complaining of pain that he was unable to diagnose accurately. He gave half of these patients, chosen randomly, a reassuring diagnosis and told them that they would get better very quickly. With the other half, he remained vague, and suggested that they come back if their pain persisted. Two weeks later, 64 per cent of the patients in the first group had improved markedly, while only 39 per cent of those in the second group had done so.
- In 2010, studies of pain showed that cognitive therapy and mindfulness training are more effective for chronic pain and depression than many treatments. These techniques have also been shown to have a physical effect on brain pathways, reversing the eroding myelination (rebuilding strong and insulated neural pathways) in the brain's grey matter.

 When undergoing surgery, there is evidence to show that the more you understand the problems of your injury/condition, how the surgery will work and the benefits you'll get, the less post-operative pain you will have and the less pain relief you will need. Understanding *less* about your condition or the procedure results in more acute pain and more medication being needed.

---

4. Taking Back Control (of Pain and of Your Life)

Having explored the nature of pain and how we experience it, let's focus on turning that knowledge into some practical steps. In this chapter, we will explore how to take control and feed your brain with evidence, so your pain becomes a more realistic reflection of your condition. We will explore overcoming skewed thinking and rumination and how you can develop optimism and resilience. You will learn more about your own pain and empowering yourself, all of which you can then use in putting together a self-management plan. But one thing to bear in mind: plans almost always fail because they don't address the most important issues properly. Take enough time to feel comfortable with the issues raised in this chapter *before* beginning your plan.

Taking Control

There is considerable evidence from healthcare organisations across the world that people with chronic conditions benefit greatly from taking responsibility for actively managing their conditions, monitoring their progress and planning their own treatments.

We have already shown, however, that for some people being encouraged to take this role on is perceived as criticism. For others, while they are coping with pain as best they can, they can be restricted by few options or little power to change things, as we saw with some of the people in the introduction. Some people also think very traditionally about the role of doctors, about what chronic pain is and the alternatives available. Fewer people understand how to self-manage chronic pain and the limitations of painkilling drugs. So, being dependent and awaiting treatment from an overstretched doctor or healthcare system leaves many feeling frustrated and even more in pain.

One important lesson we can draw from pain research is that pain affects everyone differently and that to manage it, you need a bespoke, individual plan which reflects your needs and particular situation. Another key point is that chronic pain can be modified by a range of approaches, including some, like mindfulness, relaxation or visualisation, which don't require medical expertise. In fact, many people with conditions like arthritis are told that little can be done – other than using painkillers which work less effectively over time – but we now know that boosting emotional well-being and developing positive thought processes can modify the pain they experience. This isn't flaky 'all in the mind' stuff either. We have good evidence about the physiological basis through which techniques such as stress reduction, mindfulness, cognitive behavioural therapy, gate therapy and other techniques work.

Taking control and becoming your own pain manager involves accepting that your brain controls your nervous systems and the way you perceive pain. It involves systematically monitoring the pain you get, how you react, the situations, times and context when it is worst, and how or if it changes with treatment. From that you can start to develop a personal pain management plan with simple techniques to boost your resistance and control. But taking charge of your pain and overcoming it is not simply about thinking differently, it involves *taking action* and *doing things differently*: getting and taking the right medication for you, following a healthy diet, organising regular physical health checks, seeking spiritual support or strength from relationships, and building psychological resilience and strength. Because psychological factors are so important for pain control, your frame of mind is vitally important. Your perspective, outlook and feelings of risk will also be explored in this chapter.

Questionnaire 3:
Pain Reactions Questionnaire

This questionnaire will help you to highlight the thoughts and perspectives that will both help and hinder you, either in planning to manage your pain or in relation to the motivation and resilience you need. Please don't look at the scoring instructions which follow until you have completed it.

Think about how you react when you feel pain. You will probably react differently from one day to another – that's to be expected – but to get the most from this questionnaire, you will have to think a bit more broadly. What is your reaction overall?

Here are fourteen statements about your pain. Rate each statement from 1 (meaning you never react that way) to 10 (meaning you always tend to think that). When you have completed the questionnaire, read about the issues it measures in this chapter so that the meaning of the scoring instructions will make more sense.

	Statement	Score from 1–10
1	It's terrible and I think it's never going to get any better	
2	It's awful and it just overwhelms me	
3	I worry all the time about whether the pain will ever end	
4	I feel I just can't stand it any more	
5	It makes me think I can't go on	
6	There is nothing I can do to reduce the intensity of the pain any more	
7	I am really anxious and want the pain to go away	
8	It's pretty much the first thing I think about when I wake up	
9	I keep thinking about how it hurts and what it stops me doing	
10	I can't get away from wanting the pain to stop	
11	I can't get the pain and my situation out of my mind	
12	I worry the pain will get even worse over time	
13	It makes me think of other painful experiences which I or others have had	
14	I sometimes wonder whether something serious might go wrong with me	

Scoring Your Pain Reactions Questionnaire

The Pain Reactions Scale Questionnaire (Walton, D., 2008, after Sullivan et al., 1995) was designed to assess the degree to which these elements may pose a problem for you when you develop your plans for improving your pain management. There are brief descriptions of what you are scoring here, but much more later in the chapter.

Add up your scores for the statements in these three groups, then add the three scores together for an overall picture of your reactions to pain.

- **Helplessness** (Statements 1–6):   _____
  Your subtotal will be between 6 and 60

- **Rumination** (Statements 7–11):   _____
  Your subtotal will be between 5 and 50

- **Magnification** (Statements 12–14):   _____
  Your subtotal will be between 3 and 30

- **Total score:**   _____
  Between 14 and 140

So, what do your scores mean?

When used in a clinic or session with your doctor, these scores and the rationale behind your answers can lead to a useful conversation about how significant negative and positive perspectives are for overcoming the negative effects of pain. In pain clinics, people with a **total score above 100** typically had found that their pain experience pushed them into ways of looking at their situation, described as the three aspects of your score: helplessness, rumination and magnification. These are described in much more detail later in the book, because they often cause problems for planning, getting support, and maintaining resilience and motivation – skills you need to control pain. These ways of thinking are sometimes called the depressive effect of chronic illness.

However, people may also have severe pain but a different situation and outlook – they will be less influenced by pain's depressive effects. They tend to obtain **overall scores between 60 and 100**. These are usually people for whom self-management of their chronic pain should be well within their capabilities. As with people achieving **overall scores below 60**, the pain they experience does not seem to have created the depression and hopelessness which some pain sufferers experience and which result in low motivation or the resilience needed to manage your own care or try new approaches.

One example of the depressive effect of chronic illness is catastrophising – fearing that the very worst will always happen, predicting negative futures and repeatedly being absorbed with unhelpful thoughts about the worst aspects of everything.

Catastrophising

Implementing your plans for better pain control and coping with the changes they may require is not always easy. Dealing with chronic pain, being motivated to try new things and coping with failures is challenging. But your perspective, optimism and belief in what you can achieve is vital.

In the 1980s, psychologist Aaron Beck was trying to help patients plan their recovery when he noticed that most of those having difficulty tended to catastrophise in their thinking. **Catastrophising** not only contributes to pain, emotional distress and persistent problems, but also decreases the probability that patients will take control of their pain and use new ideas to change their perception of it.

Beck suggested to them that doing this involved different things: elements of **rumination** (e.g. 'I can't stop thinking about how much it hurts'), **magnification** ('I worry that something serious may happen') and **helplessness** ('There is nothing I can do to reduce the intensity of the pain'). Over the last twenty years, repeated research studies have found these elements increase pain and diminish both resolve and resilience.

A **score of 30 or more for the rumination subscale** represents a clinically important level of catastrophising, which is likely to show in above-average negative perspectives and the avoidance of positive opportunities for change. The nature of the catastrophising tends to be one which emphasises negatives, and in clinic these patients often have difficulty reminding themselves about positive aspects of their well-being.

Looking at the balance of scores between the questionnaire's three scales will tell you about the form which your negative thinking may take. For example, a high score for magnification may represent either overestimating difficulties or underestimating your capacity to achieve things. High scores for helplessness may raise questions about the assumptions you make about yourself, your independence and self-reliance, and self-confidence/image.

Try talking over the results of this questionnaire with your family, your doctor or other health professional involved in your care, and explore how you can get support with implementing your self-management plan. In Part Two we'll explore helplessness in more detail as well as some advice about avoiding rumination.

Helplessness, rumination and magnification are unhealthy habits to get into because we almost inevitably begin to believe negative thoughts, rather than taking a more balanced view of the situation. When we're feeling depressed, we often automatically take a negative view of things, which can lead to an increased likelihood of exaggerating negatives and ignoring possibilities. We may eventually realise that the negative thought was partial or untrue but, by this time, we've already endured the anxiety and stress that it caused. Similarly, if we feel anxious, we tend to overestimate the chances of something bad happening, while also underestimating our ability to cope.

Here are five rules of thumb to limit catastrophising:

▶ Don't exaggerate. Stay specific.

One of the most common cognitive errors underlying catastrophic thinking involves exaggerating the effect of something negative, imagining that if one aspect of your life is going poorly, then your entire life is falling apart. All-or-nothing and black-and-white thinking are cousins to this mindset. When you engage in these types of thinking, it becomes less and less possible to salvage ways to be optimistic, because the whole of your perspective is being painted over with a negative brush. To change your way of thinking, start small: which aspects of your home, your daily routine, and your loved ones continue to bring you joy and comfort? Which pieces of your life still feel good to you? Which parts of your life feel safe, make you laugh, bring you pleasure, and keep you relaxed? Don't let those be tainted by thinking in overgeneralised terms.

▶ Sleep.

We all know that we feel worse when we are sleep-deprived: it often makes us more irritable and unable to think clearly. We may understand how this affects our interactions with others, but we often are less aware of how much it can distort all our thinking. There is evidence that sleep deprivation leads to becoming oversensitive to danger and risk, which stimulates our brains to be even more risk-averse towards pain. It leads us to more negative interpretations of things and as a result we turn molehills into mountains.

▶ Remember, thoughts do not define you.

Often, part of what sets a downward spiral in motion is not just our negative thoughts ('The whole world has gone to pot!'), but the fact that we're also very upset about having those thoughts in the first place ('Why do I always think like this? What is wrong with me?'). This makes for something of a double-whammy. We all have thoughts that are disturbing at times, and if we acknowledge them simply as thoughts and let them pass, we are less likely to become mired in them. I sometimes think things won't ever change and even that the world is going mad. But that's usually because of the mood I'm in. Like any thought, it will go eventually. I don't have to be someone who always thinks that way. I can choose to sit with it for the moment then watch it go away.

▶ Don't conflate the present (or the past) with the future.

Hopelessness is often a product of depression separating those who feel that life is fundamentally worth it from those who struggle to maintain that belief. It's easy to assume that because things are a certain way now, they will always be that way. Someone who has been sick for a long time may find it difficult to imagine how they'll feel when they are better. Psychologist Martin Seligman researched the idea of learned helplessness: when a person comes to believe that if they didn't have control over something at some point in the past, they will never have control over it – and shouldn't even bother to try. His recent books include *Learned Optimism* and *Authentic Happiness*; either is worth reading to get you thinking about well-being, happiness and resilience.

▶ Get physical.

Physical activities have been shown to help people reduce anxious distress in the moment. This, in part, is because they bring you into the present by helping you interact with your surroundings, which makes it harder to dwell on the past or the future. This could be getting some fresh air, chopping vegetables, going for a swim, feeling garden soil on your fingers, taking a deep breath, doing a particularly good round of stretching, taking a hot bath, hammering a nail, or feeling the soothing repetition of knitting or embroidery. If you can get to a park, see those individually changing leaves on that spectacular oak. Find whatever calms your mind, learn to value what is around you and genuinely appreciate life. You may benefit from activity-induced endorphin surges too.

Explain Pain

THINK ABOUT IT

There are many things you can do to control your pain and its effect on you. The brain controls pain, but unfortunately you are not in complete control of your brain. It's not your opinion of your injury/condition that counts, it's what your brain concludes from the evidence it gathers – and that can be instinctive rather than planned.

We now recognise that to control and diminish your pain, it is essential to develop an understanding of how pain mechanisms work (which we've explored in previous chapters) and the realities of your condition – what makes you feel personally vulnerable as well as what helps you to feel safe and in control. This goes hand in hand with getting an early diagnosis and the best advice about dealing with your condition, and agreeing a plan of management that is safe and effective for you.

Neuroscientist Lorimer Moseley and clinical educationalist David Butler are pioneers in this field and have created a programme they call 'Explain Pain', which gets pain sufferers to identify these factors. They encourage people to be aware that, with chronic pain, 'although they may be in real pain, they may not be in real danger'. Their experience is that people who think it through and keep that awareness in their daily lives can deal with pain more easily.

Both your brain and body have a remarkable capacity for renewal. Neuroplasticity is the ability to form, renew, change and discard systems in your brain (brain cells, connections and pathways). Bioplasticity is your body's capacity to do the same for nerves, muscles or tissues which are needed, underused or unnecessary. For instance, if we exercise, our muscles grow. If we practise the violin, we develop greater dexterity. If we think more, we become faster at solving problems. And if we use our minds in certain ways, we can change the way our brains use chemicals to inhibit depression, pain and other mental health problems. In short, our internal systems adapt to help us survive.

The problem is that the longer our pain system has been protecting us, the better a job it does and the more resistant to change it is. Clinical studies have shown, however, that if you understand pain and the roles of risk, or insecurity, and the roles of positive well-being and information about your situation your threshold pain can 'reset', reducing pain and discomfort. It won't happen overnight but, just as you can learn to play the cello, you can learn how to close down your protective, although discomforting, pain system.

For example, Jenny is a musician and is often disabled by pain from arthritis. But she says (both to herself and anyone who'll listen): 'I may have pain, but I'm not in danger. Or getting any worse. Or going to die. It's normal for older people who've lived active lives to have some arthritis, and I can plan how to get around it.'

Teaching yourself to do this is less demanding than you might think. It is a skill you can learn. In Part Two we'll get into this and other skills in more detail, including mindfulness and meditation.

Providing evidence for your brain to control pain means:

- Thinking differently, talking about positive things, learning about possibilities for improving, getting involved in things which make you feel good, seeing new people, and doing new and challenging things.
- Re-tuning your over-protective brain to a realistic level of danger and boosting your sense of well-being to make managing pain more possible.

Perhaps the most important thing you can do daily to improve pain is to keep in mind how your condition and the risks you face in life generally are balanced by aspects that enhance your security and well-being. Think of this as a seesaw you are teaching your brain to balance:

What risks do I face
from my condition and
in my life?

What makes me
secure and gives me
well-being in life?

with

Your approach to risk and awareness of well-being will be drawn from your experience: the places you go and people you see; things you do or say; things you think or believe; aspects of your life like your progress and hopes, or problems and fears; and the feelings or sensations you experience within your body.

Being aware of these events and how you feel about them increases your awareness of the overall level of risk or security you feel. This is what your brain considers as it manages your pain – your need to do something to protect yourself. As things change, you will have new evidence which may change the balance of risk and well-being. For instance:

- When you have financial problems and your income becomes even more stretched; your carer snaps and says, 'Stop whingeing'; you come down with another infection or think you need stronger painkillers – these are what your brain sees as *risk*.
- When your doctor tells you to try some gentle exercise because mobility will decrease pain; your friends are supportive; your boss is trying to help; you are using the knowledge you glean from this book – these are new evidence for *well-being*.

Examples of Risk
- The sound of a dentist's drill
- Looking at a worrying X-ray

- Being alone all the time
- Having so many pills to take
- Signs of degeneration and old age
- Persistent pain
- No private medical insurance
- The smell of the hospital
- Mistrust of a nosey neighbour or nurse
- Acute inflammation
- Anxiety
- Believing you might end up in a wheelchair
- A diagnosis without knowing what it means
- Someone says, 'Your pain is probably psychosomatic.'

Examples of Well-being
- Getting a clinical all-clear
- Being warm and comfortable
- Going out
- Learning about pain
- Maybe no complete solutions but at least a light at the end of the tunnel
- Confidence in the doctor and the information they provide
- Going to a café after a hospital appointment
- Liking the nurse
- Optimism
- New medication
- Awareness of scientifically proven path to recovery
- Going to a self-help group for people with pain
- Getting listed for spinal cord stimulation

This balancing framework works on the premise that the brain reacts to perceptions of risk and threat at an unconscious level, changing the intensity and level of pain we perceive and that, ultimately, *everything that provides evidence of risk or well-being can influence the pain we feel.* When risk outweighs well-being, your brain concludes the balance of evidence means it needs to further stimulate your nervous systems, making them more sensitive and aware of anything which might be a further risk. If well-being outweighs risk, stress and anxiety are less likely to affect your thinking, and the stimulation of your nervous systems will be maintained at your normal levels.

 Use your notebook to make two lists of your own – risk factors and well-being factors affecting you now. Use the examples shown above to prompt your thinking, and make both lists real and current.

Pain Gateways

By now we should be agreed that the way in which we experience pain is very complex. For example, you will probably have experienced times when, even though you have pain, you are only dimly aware of it. This can happen when you are really engrossed in something interesting or dealing with a situation which demands all your attention. On the other hand, you will probably be aware of circumstances in which your pain feels worse the more you think about it. One way to understand what is happening here is **Pain Gate Control** – a helpful way of making sense of our pain experience.

As we discussed earlier, our peripheral and central nervous systems pick up information about danger or risk to our cells and pass it, via the spinal cord, to the brain. The first main meeting point for the nervous systems is in the spine's 'dorsal horn', where a complex interaction occurs between signals going to the brain then back to peripheral nerves, and special cells called 'interneurons', activated by neurotransmitters from the brain. Only a theory in 1965, Ronald Melzack and Patrick Wall's ideas about pain gates have prompted recent research to identify the mechanisms involved, and to explain how nerve and brain functions are linked, thereby explaining both the physical and psychological aspects of pain perception.

A good way to visualise this is to imagine a series of gates (nerve groups which have special sensitivities) in the spine, where messages about pain arrive from the body on their way up to and back from the brain, down through your body. These gates are normally partly open, but they open more fully when the brain senses damage. The opening and closing of the gates are managed by the interneurons referred to above, which act as gatekeepers. Opening allows more signals through to the brain, and you are likely to experience a higher level of pain. If the gates are more closed, then fewer messages get through, and you are likely to experience less pain.

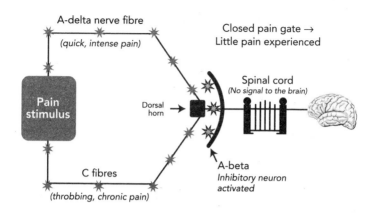

© Cognitive Escape Network

Opening Pain Gateways

There are three main factors that influence when the gates open and close, which can be divided into sensory, emotional and cognitive influences:

- **Sensory**: One of the most important categories is how information coming from your senses is received and responded to by the brain. Because of a process called bioplasticity – the way our bodies change to meet new circumstances – our whole bodies, including our nerves, adapt to meet new challenges. Nerves can become more sensitive. New connections grow in the brain to deal with new information. So, when people with chronic pain move around less, have stiffer joints and lack fitness, it encourages pain gates to both open and stay open, allowing a more constant flow of signals (along C fibres), which reinforces the pain. This is not simply the pain of stiff joints but permanent changes (oversensitivity to senses) that make us feel pain more easily.

- **Emotional**: Stress, anxiety, worry, anger, depression and tension can all lead to the gates to pain being more open. Tension is a common gate opener and one of the most effective ways of increasing your pain; it leads to focusing all your attention on it. Anxiety and boredom can also create conditions where this happens.

- **Cognitive**: When we have a negative frame of mind we look for things that are wrong – resulting in a greater perception of, and focus on, discomfort, risk or threat. Being on autopilot and reacting emotionally without any counterbalance results in open gateways and a greater pain experience. (Cognitive behavioural therapy and pain management are tools which can help avoid both this and similar 'thinking problems' which can make pain worse. We will look at the principles behind them later.)

Closing Pain Gateways

When the interneurons close the gates, their function is 'inhibitory', closing off the stimulus used by the brain to create pain. Inhibitory interneurons can be activated in several ways:

- **Physical soothing activity** – like touching, rubbing, gentle stroking, cooling or warming – encourages the brain to activate the inhibitory gatekeepers, therefore reducing the perception of pain. Activation happens when neurotransmitters like serotonin and gamma-aminobutyric acid are dispersed to calm the central nervous system.
- **Conscious thought**: Awareness of general well-being, safety and practical plans for overcoming any pain-causing conditions will enable the frontal cortex, working in concert with the emotional centre of the brain (amygdala), to trigger neurotransmitters which calm the central nervous system, and enable the inhibitory response at the pain gates. Mindfulness and cognitive behavioural and pain management techniques are useful, but knowing what affects your well-being and safety is essential. (For a pain gate exercise, see page 165.)
- **Spinal cord stimulation**: There are also mechanical means to activate pain gates. A spinal cord stimulator consists of a small computer (matchbox-sized) placed under the skin in your abdomen or chest that controls an electrode near your spine. Tiny electrical charges are then sent to your spinal cord. The electrode stimulates, among other nerves, the inhibitory interneuron described earlier. If the spinal cord stimulator is successful, you feel tingling instead of pain in the part of your body that normally hurts. Some people seem more sensitive to this than others.

Pain and the Importance of Your Perspective

Many people feel that being in pain, having restricted movement and perhaps feeling cut off from social activities severely dent their sense of confidence and empowerment. What about you? Do you believe you have power to create opportunities and to influence what happens, or the responsibility for successes and failures? Consider the situations of two people with similar spinal and joint pain from osteoarthritis:

Person A

- Feels unable to go on holiday with the family
- Thinks few people can be bothered to spend time with 'disabled people'
- Watches a lot of television
- Thinks surgery will solve the problem
- Checks the house is locked three times before leaving to catch the bus
- Is scared about what their future holds.

Person B

- Organises the family holiday
- Has volunteered to work with an arthritis charity when possible
- Reads a newspaper every day and goes to a book club
- Is a passionate supporter of community and workers' rights
- Thinks eating better will help solve the problem
- Is scared about the future the grandchildren will have.

THINK ABOUT IT

1. Which person is likely to have the more negative outlook and why? How might they differ in the way they cope with their pain?
2. Now look at the conversations which they had about pain with their doctors: how will their subsequent outlook and behaviour differ?

Person A sees Doctor A, who says:

'OK, you've damaged your back lifting at work. The X-ray you had yesterday shows very early osteoarthritis; rest if it hurts too much. Your pain is a warning that you've overdone things. It can only get worse with age; there is no cure for arthritis.'

Person B sees Doctor B, who says:

'Your pain is due to an acute soft tissue sprain. The body has tremendous powers of healing; it's a self-limiting problem. No real harm has been done; keep as active as you can within the pain, and then you will have a 90 per cent chance of it all settling down on its own without treatment in a few weeks or months at the very worst.'

Doctors A and B have different views about how they should help patients and the extent to which people can help themselves or should rely on doctors. They have unwittingly instilled different beliefs into the patients' minds which may reinforce some of their natural tendencies. In practice, these two patients dealt with their back pain very differently. What do you think the differences might have been?

Person A developed a negative set of beliefs around age, their back pain, expecting that they were doomed forever and that it could only get worse. Because they believe they have been 'told by their doctor', they will fit the dependent patient role: they will now modify their behaviour, become less active, develop more back pain because of their inactivity, and slowly spiral downwards into disability, pain and dependency. But there are more problems in store for Patient A.

These beliefs are also inadvertently reinforced by loved ones and colleagues at work when they may be overly concerned about the pain and encourage Person A always to take it easy.

When they link the pain to every movement, Person A thinks that the back has been damaged further and the pain seems to get worse. Several things then begin to happen:

- They become frightened to do anything that may cause the pain – this is called **anticipatory anxiety**. They anticipate the pain before they move, causing them to hold their breath and guard their back, while tightening their back muscles. This increases the pain during movement, as most of the pain is muscular in the first place.

- The mood of the person worsens over time with a tendency to 'catastrophise' about the pain, its cause and its consequences. (Turning pain from a natural ageing condition into a catastrophe increases anxiety and the likelihood it will seem worse than it actually is.) Whenever they think about why this has happened, the pain becomes worse again.
- They tend to misinterpret the severity of the pain, leading to a vicious spiral downwards into depression.

When Person A eventually presents to a pain clinic for help, they have firmly entrenched views about the severity of the pain, its cause and their need for surgery as the only solution.

THINK ABOUT IT What could Person A and their doctor have done differently to manage their case better?

Person B developed positive beliefs around their back pain, expecting that the pain would go away on its own, and that maintaining normal activities would be good therapy. It is quite likely that this person will recover fully and go on to have a normal lifestyle. They are likely to think positively about the causes of their pain.

Back pain can result from many causes:
- Years of poor posture
- Sleeping on a poor mattress
- Poor safety habits when lifting or carrying heavy objects
- Being overweight, which can put strain on the back and legs
- Congenital conditions
- Traumatic injury and ineffective healing
- Wearing inappropriate footwear – particularly unsupportive shoes or high heels
- Insufficient stretching, exercise and general mobility.

But sometimes, there is simply no obvious physical cause.

Fatigue and Anxiety

Pain is often accompanied by unrelenting fatigue and low mood. Both will fluctuate in their intensity, but sometimes people feel isolated or angry that life isn't what they expected it to be. A resulting sense of loss makes it difficult to accept the realities of the situation. Often people in these circumstances tend to think a lot about the past rather than tackling their current situation and any issues which cause difficulty.

Asking others for help isn't always easy, especially if you are worried about being a burden or take pride in your independence. If you are finding the physical or psychological effect of your pain too much, it's time for action.

The truth is, everyone needs help at some time, and most people will try to help you become and stay independent, if that's what you want.

People who reject help from others frequently find that depression and anxiety start to overwhelm them, and both are common in people with pain. We all can feel low for a while, but depression is different. It goes on for weeks or perhaps months, interfering with your daily life in many ways. Motivation suffers, and any sense of enjoyment can be lost. Hopelessness is common, with sleeplessness compounding the problem. It's often accompanied by anxiety, constant worry or a feeling of vulnerability. Some people cope by becoming isolated, cold and distant, others by becoming cynical or negative even about small, everyday things. Some become aggressive, particularly towards people who are trying to help. Each of these can be a risk factor for depression, made worse by a lack of empowerment, the ability to change things. Depression can be managed and gradually lifted, but long-term improvement is almost always linked to feeling more in control and acquiring the confidence and power to challenge the situation, ask for help if needed and achieve (sometimes very small) positive changes.

Because mind and body are so closely linked, your pain and the emotions you feel will influence one another. For example, being in pain and being unable to move easily can make you short-tempered or unhappy. On the other hand, feeling good about finding a way to achieve something and being focused on what you *can* do makes the bodily sensations easier to handle.

Rest, relaxation and sleep are important elements of becoming self-empowered and avoiding depression. Pain makes most people anxious, and the body's physical response to stress can make that anxiety and insecurity worse. You can handle the long-term physical effects of stress and create a calm and purposeful approach to your pain. It involves learning to relax, pacing yourself (resting between effort and activity) and getting sleep. We will look at practical suggestions for improving relaxation and sleep patterns in Part Two.

THINK ABOUT IT

Pain Clinics
One striking feature of pain clinics is the boost which people get from hearing others discussing their approach for dealing with common problems. Being with others in similar situations and seeing their perspectives, strength of mind and confidence is helpful – but something of a challenge if your pain has left you feeling that you can't cope. However, most people find that if a clinic is available to them, their outlook on pain management becomes more positive and the practical help and experience of others is extremely valuable. Clinics look at practical, traditional and non-traditional treatments and help develop personal pain management plans, although some do focus more on medication, dosage and prescribing.

Others follow a widely used agenda of topics, which you might like to learn more about:

- Nerves and how they work in the body
- Medicines and the best way to manage them
- Becoming fitter and more active
- Using pacing to help reduce severe pain levels
- Setting physical, emotional and lifestyle goals
- Resolving problems in day-to-day living
- Rewarding yourself and positive self-talk
- Maintaining positive changes
- Talking through difficulties with relationships/others
- Mood and emotional disturbance
- Relaxation skills – breathing, imagery, sounds, meditation.

Having read this book, you might find learning further about these topics will help you to develop your own pain management plan. In the same way that knowing about your medical condition empowers you to ask questions and make decisions, knowing more about how others are using pain management gives you options.

Skewed Thinking

Pain, stress, anxiety and depression frequently appear together when people suffer pain. We tend to think that the pain is the main problem, but it is usually only the beginning. Illness and isolation can lead to changes in how we think, creating patterns which can persist or become automatic reactions. These forms of thinking, including 'catastrophising', 'rumination' and 'learned helplessness', tend to be negative and make the world seem very dark and threatening; they have several consequences, described in the following sections. They affect the personal empowerment, resilience, optimism and motivation needed for coping with chronic pain.

You can often detect closed or 'bunkered' thinking, even hopelessness, in how people use language, their attitudes and the assumptions they make. Their thinking often becomes less positive and more judgemental, often seeking oversimplified solutions.

Periods of isolation, poor health, chronic pain and depression create cognitive changes: different patterns of perception, analysis and decision making. Ten ways in which thinking and decision making can change are shown below; these have been identified in people who have unresolved healthcare problems. Relationships, social contacts, wellbeing and mental health can all be adversely affected. The cognitive changes we describe as 'skewed thinking' might lead to blowing things out of proportion, misunderstanding, miscommunication, relationship problems, reinforcing a negative frame of mind and being unaware of opportunities for improvement. Many people fall into the trap of thinking this way from time to time, particularly about finding better ways to live with pain if it can't be cured.

Asking questions like 'Am I looking at this in the right way?' or 'What's influencing the view I'm taking?' and 'Is it the only way of seeing things?' are useful to make sure we are being realistic about the situation and making sure the most important issues are considered and resolved.

 Some might think there is no likelihood of controlling their pain (all-or-nothing thinking) or that they only feel better because someone else has looked after them (disqualifying positives). Perhaps they are worried about discussing medical issues with a doctor (emotional reasoning) or that their hip pain or movement will lead to the hip fragmenting (magnification and catastrophising).

You may know people who seem like this. Read the descriptions below and think about what skewed thinking they might be showing.

Black-and-White (All-or-Nothing) Thinking, e.g.

- Thinking that if we don't get perfect solutions we have failed
- There is no nuance, only right or wrong
- There's only one way of looking at things

Mental Filtering

- Only one thing is important
- Can see what's wrong but with no awareness of what's right
- Can see risk but not safety

Jumping to Conclusions
- Not taking account of all the information
- Imagining we know what others think
- Treating guesses about the future as fact

Emotional Reasoning
- Rationalising what we think to fit how we feel
- Assuming whatever we think must be true

Labelling
- Thinking in stereotypes
- Thinking 'I'm useless' or 'They just don't care'
- Thinking 'I'm no doctor, so I can't plan my own care'

Overgeneralising
- Drawing conclusions based on a single event or limited evidence
- Being overly broad in our conclusions: 'They *all* must …'

Disqualifying the Positive
- Discounting good things or achievements
- Not looking for the upside
- Thinking problems are more important than achievements

Magnifying (Catastrophising) and Minimising
- Blowing things out of proportion
- Denying the importance of particular issues

- Pretending some issues are insignificant, to deny their importance

Using Critical, Guilt-provoking Words
- Using words like 'should', 'must' and 'ought' suggests failure
- Implying someone else is responsible
- Taking views which may not recognise practical constraints

Personalisation
- Attributing blame to individuals
- Blaming ourselves for something not completely our fault
- Blaming others for our actions

Catastrophic Thinking
One particularly important category of skewed thinking is catastrophising: where someone is so concerned about an issue that it becomes central to their whole aware-ness; it becomes so important that facts and information are sidelined because of the emotional impact they may have. Sometimes the product of an overactive imagination (although more often a result of anxiety or depression), catastrophising is a cognitive distortion which makes an unpleasant and undesirable situation worse than it really is, or need be.

CASE STUDY

It's 4pm on a Thursday afternoon. My twelve-year-old daughter should have been home from school half an hour ago, but she's nowhere to be seen.

The pessimist in me thinks that she rarely remembers to ring if something comes up, but after two hours, my mind leaps to the worst-case scenario. She has been knocked off her bike by a bus, and is lying at the side of the road, unconscious. I hear an ambulance siren in the distance and my heart rate skyrockets. It's surely only a matter of time before the police knock at my door.

Pessimists (or realists, as they like to call themselves) tend to expect failure and worry about whether it will happen. Catastrophising involves an exaggerated bad response to a situation, and the belief that this result is inevitable. (I might have denied it later, but at the time, I really worried she might have died!)

Two minutes after the sirens pass, my daughter bursts in, dumping her bag on the mat. 'Sorry I'm late,' she pants. 'My bike chain came off.' Relief overwhelms me as I realise that I've been catastrophising – a thought pattern that we are drawn into, all too easily, the more anxious we are.

Catastrophising is a form of thinking in which a person instinctively thinks the worst about a situation, speculates about why it has happened and fears what may come next.

Triggered by circumstances, emotional states and experiences, it's negative *automatic* thinking which can affect all aspects of life, reinforcing worry, anxiety and depression. The idea of catastrophic thinking was refined by psychologist Aaron Beck in 1987; it came to his notice originally with patients with anxiety and depressive disorders with an irrational negative forecast of future events.

Nearly 600 studies have been published documenting the link between catastrophising and pain. These have included patients with rheumatoid arthritis, osteoarthritis, fibromyalgia, sickle cell disease, soft tissue injuries and neuropathic pain, as well as dental patients and patients recovering from surgery. The research suggests that, even for people with previously good mental health, the hopelessness they can experience, alongside a lack of positive medical outcomes and isolation, encourages them to catastrophise. According to recent studies, catastrophising diminishes their motivation to be proactive and to manage their own pain. It has been demonstrated with groups of children as young as seven years old.

Catastrophising may have some positive value, however, with research emerging to show that individuals who catastrophise are more aware of pain signals and can express their current physical and emotional distress more easily. This could help early detection of more serious problems, as other people may only understand what help is needed if distress is clearly expressed. However, the productive value of catastrophising is greatly outweighed by evidence of the problems it creates.

THINK ABOUT IT A famous example of catastrophic thinking is that of Mexican painter Frida Kahlo. In the 1940s, she was badly injured, resulting in horrific treatments and unbearable neuropathic pain and fibromyalgia. Her own diaries and interviews and reports of friends show that, while maintaining her painting, her life was full of unhappiness and pain. The catastrophe occupying her mind was portrayed within a series of surrealistic paintings centred around the theme of brokenness and hopelessness. An undoubtedly talented artist, catastrophising had the effect of making those themes a central issue for her, with a negative effect on her relationships, perspective and many practical aspects of the way she lived.

Research among patients with work-related upper limb disorders and severe pain shows that catastrophising is a predictor for how long pain is experienced and overall recovery outcomes. Similarly, catastrophising patients with musculoskeletal pain showed lack of improvement and continued disability compared to other patients. Most studies, including those of back, shoulder, neck, cancer or arthritic conditions, have consistently highlighted pain catastrophising as a predictor for poor recovery and emotional stability, affecting both acute injury and pain conditions.

Patients who tend to catastrophise are often helped by cognitive behavioural therapy (CBT), which treats negative automatic thinking as a prime concern. You can read more on this in Part Two, but you might like to try the following preliminary CBT activity to establish whether it should be a priority for you.

 Use the ABC Worksheet below to identify the effects of a recent painful episode. Think of a time during the last week or so when your chronic pain has been very bad.

What follows is a sample worksheet from someone with very serious pain, followed by a blank worksheet for you to use.

The worksheet will ask you to identify the ABC of the episode: the Activating event, your Beliefs and automatic thoughts at the time, and the Consequences. When you have completed the worksheet, review the Beliefs and Consequences columns to assess whether, in hindsight, your reactions were stronger than you think are appropriate, whether more information might have influenced your reactions, and whether the beliefs they were based on could be modified.

The ABC Worksheet (sample)

Activating Event Serious Pain Situation	Beliefs Automatic Reactions and Thoughts	Consequences Emotional, Physical and Behavioural
Tuesday morning Moved over in bed and had an agonisingly sharp hip pain followed by aching legs and back. Couldn't move for fifteen minutes.	Every movement means a pain so bad I don't think I can cope. Why me? What did I do to deserve this? I'm in for a miserable few days.	E: Made me cry. Frustrated and angry P: Legs are swollen and hot, shooting pains down my muscles/tendons B: Don't move so I don't cause more pain
Tuesday afternoon Stayed in chair all morning. Any movement excruciating. Took largest dose of painkillers but little effect. Grandchildren visited.	It feels worse than being stuck. I sometimes think my life is over. I love my grandchildren but I wish they'd come next week. Don't want them to see granny screaming when the tablets wear off.	E: Close to the end of my tether P: Getting to the loo so difficult I wet myself. Whole body seems to throb and can't stand any noise B: Just cry all the time

97

The ABC Worksheet (sample)

Activating Event Serious Pain Situation	Beliefs Automatic Reactions and Thoughts	Consequences Emotional, Physical and Behavioural

Rumination – Getting Lost in Our Thoughts, Anxieties and Memories

Thinking about problems is, without doubt, part of how we solve them. If we need to deal with one of our life issues, we think it through, review our various options, and then choose a course of action. A bit of introspection, positive reflection and self-challenge can help us take appropriate action. But when mulling things over goes wrong, it can make us feel stuck and less inclined actually to do anything constructive about the situation and our associated distress. The deeper we get in a cycle of overthinking, the harder it can be to recognise that it's happening and to dig our way out.

Sometimes the effect of pain draws us into constantly dwelling on our difficulties, worries and why they are happening. We might repeatedly think about events from our past or become constantly preoccupied with questions ('How can I cope with the pain') which we have neither answer for, nor can get out of our minds. This repetitive and involuntary overthinking is **rumination**; usually driven by anxiety, it tends to focus on *causes* rather than *solutions*, is *speculative* rather than *evidence-based*, and usually involves a *negative outlook*. Researchers have found that women are much more likely to ruminate than men and pain sufferers more than those with other health problems.

It is said that a trouble shared is a troubled halved, and extensive research confirms that being open about health concerns will reduce your own anxiety and stress. However, it can sometimes become a slippery slope towards another danger – that of **co-rumination**. People often believe that talking problems over with others will help them find answers and make them feel better. But focusing on problems and negative emotion together can increase negative beliefs and moods – particularly among younger women – and can result in a greater need for more rumination. In research findings across Europe, the USA and Australasia, co-rumination has been found to increase anxiety and depression, with a greater potential for creating stress and burnout in work settings too.

When we ruminate individually, we employ three types of skewed thinking:

- *Victimisation* – When we feel that we have been treated badly, by fate or by individuals, we ruminate about the injustice we have experienced. We review the situation again and again and think of ways we can find retribution. We don't look at the whole situation or try to understand our part in the interaction. Unfortunately, we may act on thoughts which have negative consequences.
- *Magnifying* – When we feel upset, we start thinking of reasons to explain our feelings. We may come up with many reasons, all equally plausible, although some may be overly dramatic and not grounded in reality. We can then take rash actions with negative consequences,

such as quitting our job, ending a friendship, or acting out our bad mood.

- *Chaos* – Sometimes we feel overwhelmed and our thoughts switch quickly from one focus to another; we end up feeling disoriented, and we may shut down or run away from our problems.

Rumination isn't productive thinking. It's not the same as worry, although ruminators do worry. Worry is forward looking and involves 'What if' thinking – wondering about things that might happen ('What if I say the wrong thing at work?' 'What if this date goes wrong?').

Rumination, on the other hand, focuses more on things that have happened in the past – like why an accident happened, why you get the amount of pain you do, what you meant when you said something, or why something went wrong. It is about dwelling on problems rather than on the actions required to solve them.

How Do We Overcome Rumination?

You will find the information from Questionnaire 3 (Pain Reactions Questionnaire, page 63) useful now, along with your specific scores for rumination. If it's something you are prone to do, the tips in this section will help you to avoid the rumination trap. Remember that, while rumination is an instinctive response to anxiety, it is not a healthy resolution to problems, and it may prevent you from improving your pain control or developing a positive frame of mind.

Instead of internal reflection – which can create tunnel vision and lead to depression, more anxiety and anger – talk things out with a realistic and questioning friend, and focus on action rather than on rehashing the issues and seeking fault or blame. What, where, when and who are the basic tenets of problem solving. Remember that when organisations and systems don't deliver, it's often the processes they use which are to blame. Railing at healthcare service providers may vent some frustration, but cool and specific questioning brings results.

Rumination can be a private experience and many people would not wish to share the thoughts they harbour with other people – although we have seen that this may not be true for younger people with a different attitude to social media and for many, particularly younger, women (see co-rumination above). There is evidence that a major driver for rumination is anticipatory anxiety – in which individuals speculate about people's motives and what the future might hold. Without a firm hold on basic information about the situation, their thinking may have little basis in the real world. With this specifically in mind, sharing your thoughts with an informed friend, family member or therapist can help to turn thoughts into spoken practicality and meet the challenge of explaining worries rationally and clearly. The very best therapists are informed, clear thinking and trustworthy. These are the qualities which will help you move from rumination into problem solving and action planning.

Your friend can ask relevant questions, such as 'How were you feeling when this started – what happened? How do you know that?', and their thoughts and your questions to them will allow you to see your issues in a new light. Just make sure that the person you talk to is trusted and stable. If you choose a person who simply fans the flames of your worries, you will accomplish nothing and may drift further into rumination.

Let's look at some further ways to replace the old ruminative pattern with more positive approaches. They might take time to master, and you might find help from a professional therapist or tutor beneficial, particularly if rumination is significant for you.

- **Avoid the triggers** – Learn to identify the situations that lead to rumination – and to avoid them. For example, if spending time with a particular friend leads to overthinking, you might find others to be with at times of difficulty. You might see this friend with others present perhaps or try to arrange your meetings in places where rumination would not feel appropriate (new, public, busy or noisy places, as an example).
- **Let go of unrealistic goals** – Learn to assess whether your hopes and goals are realistic or not in order to limit anxiety and tension. Goals that can't be accomplished become sources of frustration; redefining them into goals which can be accomplished reduces the need for rumination.

- ***Indulge yourself in different ways*** – Instead of going into ruminative thought when you feel stressed, learn alternate approaches. Relaxation or diversion are useful, but activities like physical exercise, massage, a bubble bath, talking with a trusted friend, nature walks, prayer or meditation are different. They trigger neurotransmitters involved in the dopamine pathways of the brain's limbic system, providing respite and well-being (although perhaps temporarily).

- ***Develop your narrative*** – Reviewing your life can provide insights and different perspectives during times of stress. Working on your narrative with a therapist can lead to a permanent change in your approach to life's challenges. Using mindfulness or meditation can help you to independently review your life and implement the changes you want.

- ***Expand your range of activities*** – Rumination is more likely to occur when our lives are limited. If your pain has taken over your life, see if voluntary or paid work is within your capabilities. Getting out and about is important and can develop your interests and social circle.

- ***Define your life in positives, not negatives*** – Rumination thrives when we see ourselves in negative terms. Learn to change the negative interpretations of your life into positives; instead of focusing on failures in your life, highlight the successes.

Co-rumination

People are not always supportive when someone comes to them with a problem, particularly if they talk about the same problem a lot. So, when would you want to share or avoid sharing your worries with others?

- **Is it problem solving?** If you find yourself talking about the same experiences over and over again – particularly those that involve difficult emotions, like anger, sadness or envy – speculating on motives and focusing on blame, it can turn into co-rumination. The more this type of discussion is repeated, the greater the risk of damaging your relationships, harming recovery and emphasising negative risks in the lives of co-ruminators.
- **Is it negative?** Recognise which topics are likely to lead to rehashing negative experiences and try to direct the focus towards tangible issues you can act on. What is the current situation and who needs to do what to improve it?
- **Avoid taking on others' problems.** Co-rumination has the potential to do real harm to people with chronic pain. People who have little knowledge of the condition can offer sympathy, and discussions with them can provide an opportunity to clarify aspects of the problem. Discussions with others sharing the same condition can be more valuable, sharing information and possible

actions to improve pain management. But in this situation, group membership can transfer others' fears to you, groundlessly.

- **Keep a balance of discussion.** Disclosure and seeking support are helpful, but in the long run, co-rumination isn't actually all that helpful for well-being or even for the problem itself. It has the potential to drive certain people away, especially when conversations tend to be overly focused on one person's difficulties or life.

- **Have a range of coping strategies.** If you try to minimise your tendency to co-ruminate, without coming up with other, more constructive ways of coping, you will likely feel overwhelmed and lonely. That's why it's equally important to find new ways to cope with whatever problem you're facing. Develop a sustainable self-care routine, and maintain a range of people to engage with. Stay with your problem-solving focus, working through the pros and cons of possible solutions, and turn to healthy distractions when all else fails.

Learned Helplessness and Optimism

In 1965, US psychologist Martin Seligman and his colleagues were researching **classical conditioning**, how animals or humans associate one thing with another. Their studies showed that animals which had received light electric shocks began to anticipate receiving other shocks. Seligman and his team went on to experiment with dogs (which had been through the first experiment), putting them in large crates that were divided down the middle by a low barrier. The dog could see and jump over the fence if necessary. The floor on one side of the fence was electrified, but the floor on the other side was not. Seligman put each dog into the crate on the electrified side and administered a light shock. He expected the dogs to jump to the non-shocking side of the fence. Instead, the dogs lay down. It was as though they'd learned from the first part of the experiment that there was nothing they could do to avoid the shocks.

 If you want to see the principle of classical conditioning in more detail, go to YouTube and search for 'Learned Helplessness and Optimism (Seligman)'.

Seligman described this conditioning as **learned helplessness**, accepting a negative situation because the past has taught you to think you have no power to affect the outcome. The phenomenon is often seen in people who have long experienced pain, helplessness to change things and reliance on medication for relief. Feeling unable to avoid the pain, they may have been unable to control events in the past or, having tried unsuccessfully, they may have given up. Further research has shown that learned helplessness comes about because of the way in which people view negative events (their thinking styles) and how much control they try to exercise (whether they accept that sometimes it may be necessary to learn to live with unsatisfactory situations). We also refer to these attitudes and behaviours as 'pessimism'. Pessimists tend to believe that bad events will last a long time, will undermine everything they do and think, and that, somehow, they are to blame.

By contrast, we might experience **learned optimism** – this reflects a fundamental difference in people's outlook. Optimists tend to believe that problems and circumstances like pain are simply temporary, that each situation should be dealt with on its own merits, and that the causes of problems are challenges rather than a fait accompli.

The different effects of these two ways of thinking are shown in hundreds of studies. Pessimists tend to resign themselves more easily and get depressed more often. Optimists do much better, demonstrating their ability to think analytically and influence others effectively. Their health is unusually good, they age well and recover from health problems both more quickly and more comprehensively. Evidence suggests they may even live longer.

In general, optimists have a sense of confidence about the future. They expect that the outcomes of particular situations are likely to be positive. Pessimists, on the other hand, have a sense of doubt and hesitancy with an expectation of negative outcomes. So, for pain, is it better to be an optimist or a pessimist?

Research has shown many advantages for optimistic viewpoints, including:

- Optimists experience less distress, anxiety and depression than pessimists when dealing with difficulties in their lives, and as a result find pain easier to cope with.
- Optimists adapt better to serious negative events like coronary surgery, breast cancer or bone marrow transplants and recover more quickly.
- Optimism creates the capability to learn from pain. It allows problem-centred coping, humour, planning and, when the situation cannot be controlled, accepting reality and working with it.
- Surprisingly, optimists avoid denial, while pessimists tend to separate themselves from the problem. Optimists don't ignore bad news, avoid 'sticking their heads in the sand' and recognise real issues which need to be dealt with. Pessimists are usually uncomfortable with the reality of problem solving and the compromise.
- Optimists exert more continuous effort and tend not to give up. Pessimists, anticipating (what they describe as) disaster, give up sooner.
- In the workplace, optimists are more productive, both in terms of forming better relationships and delivering higher output.

Avoiding Learned Helplessness

Psychologists working on learned helplessness say it is an instinctive response to lessons we have learned, rather than a matter of personal weakness. People faced with chronic pain may feel they have no influence or control and may well give up hope after trying to improve it unsuccessfully. Now we know that becoming motivated to change our situations requires us to *think and behave differently*.

Three key ideas underpin our ability to develop resilience and control:

- **Self-efficacy** involves believing in your ability to go through the steps necessary to produce a desired outcome. For example, if you want to run a marathon, you'll have to run consistently, eat right and follow through on stretching and strength building to keep yourself injury-free. If you believe that you can do all those things, then you have a high self-efficacy.
- **Locus of control** is whether you believe that you can have a significant impact on a situation. People who have tried to manage their pain using some of the ideas this book is based upon – and who have felt the benefits – have an **internalised locus**, whereas people who believe that pain and their thinking process are not connected have an **externalised locus**. The latter depend on others to improve the situation (through drugs or assistance) or convince themselves that nothing they can do themselves will help and the pain will never be manageable.

- **Being in a state of 'flow'** is about being fully involved and focused, such that you are not even aware of yourself or of time passing. Discovered and developed by Hungarian-American psychologist Mihaly Csikszentmihalyi, the idea is typified by time passing without you noticing and you becoming really charged up, empowered by concentrating on an outcome you are trying to achieve. Most people can recall being in such a state; in fact 90 per cent easily recognise it in association with particular activities. Athletes call it 'being in the zone', others a 'heightened state of consciousness' or total involvement.

From Apathy to Flow

Identify activities which get you into a state of flow – in which you become absorbed, time flies and you show some of your real talents. They could be leisure or cultural interests, charity work, your job, developing business ideas, socialising, researching or helping children to play and develop.

Reallocate time to these activities by reducing how much time you spend on 'apathetic' activities – those which often result in boredom or indifference (such as watching daytime TV, doing housework or idling) – or on anxiety issues (like spending a large portion of the day talking about pain or your health concerns).

Empowerment and Confidence

Research has shown that people who feel empowered tend to be happier, less depressed and less stressed. Psychologists call this having an internalised locus of control – feeling in control of your own destiny. Empowered people have been found to cope with pain and the effects of disabilities more easily. They are people who don't take things for granted and are prepared to question the conditions causing their pain. They are more likely to have ideas and determination and to seek out resources and sources of help.

 If you feel a lack of confidence or power to achieve things, here are some ideas to consider:

1. Realise that you always have a chance to change your situation. Even if you don't like the options available now, or even if the only change you can make is in your attitude, you always have some choice.
2. When you feel trapped, make a list of all possible courses of action. Just brainstorm and write things down without evaluating them first.
3. Talk with a friend to come up with more ideas that you may not have initially considered. Don't shoot down new ideas right away; just write them down.
4. Then, evaluate each one and decide on the best course of action for you, and keep the others in the back of your

mind as alternative options. After following this process for a while, seeing and weighing up new possibilities will become more of a habit. Notice the language you use most of the time and how you are thinking. If you tend to make lots of judgements, be careful because negative thinking can become an automatic perspective. If this describes you, CBT or mindfulness can be helpful for turning negative events and thoughts into something more positive (see the resources section at the end of the book).

5. Phase out phrases like 'I have no choice' and 'I can't ...' Replace them with 'I choose not to' or 'I don't like my choices, but I will ...'

 Realising that you always have a choice (even if the options aren't ideal) can help you to change your situation, or to accept it more easily if it really is the best of all available options.

PART TWO
Becoming Your Own Pain Manager

So, having looked at what pain is and the mechanisms which are involved, it is now time to explore the focus for your own pain management plan and how to use the ideas we've covered.

Chapter 5 gives you a framework for thinking about your own situation, your pain and how you can handle it. It involves two important tools: a pain diary and a self-management 'wheel' – a template covering what you can build into your plan. This chapter also includes ideas about planning and setting goals for you to think about.

Chapter 6 covers the emotional and cognitive issues which may affect putting your plan into action; **Chapters 7** and **8** draw on pain control ideas that chronic pain patients have found useful.

These suggestions aren't exhaustive, nor explore every-thing in the fields they introduce. To discover more about them, there are a wide range of books and leaflets produced by charities, local groups (people sharing their experiences), volunteers and healthcare organisations which all promote self-management of chronic conditions. The internet can be a great source of information, although using websites with professional and national links might help you to avoid poorly researched advice. There are some references for **Further Reading** at the end of the book.

5. Developing Your Pain Control Self-management Plan

Part One of the book was designed to give you the basis of developing your plan for taking control of your pain and your ability to manage it yourself, with the support and help of those around you. It drew on ideas which have been useful for other people who have experienced severe pain and begun to manage it successfully. Hopefully, by now you will have gained a better understanding of your pain and have begun to think about what your self-management plan could achieve. This part of the book is about preparing your plan, anticipating problems, thinking about your priorities and setting yourself some improvement goals.

But before putting the plan into action, discuss it with your doctor to ensure that anything you want to try is safe for you. One word of caution here: the information and ideas in this book are understood and shared by most specialists in pain management; however, not *all* clinicians (in particular those busy with general practice) know about or are sympathetic to these approaches. Some may not distinguish between acute and chronic pain. Others may not prioritise time to discuss chronic pain because it is rarely life-threatening. So be aware of this when talking these things over with general practice doctors; be as specific as you can and, if necessary, explore options for specialist care. Good doctors always try to make time available but, to help them, plan your conversation. Try to identify a list of key issues you want their help on, being as specific as possible.

THINK ABOUT IT

Do you need to know more about the condition causing the pain? Do you need to know more about your options for treatment? Does your doctor know the patterns of pain you experience? Are there any imminent risks of the condition getting worse? What are the advantages or risks of more exercise, and what forms might be most useful? Is diet important? Are there groups you could join to discuss your pain plans?

Try to think what your options might be beforehand. Be clear what you want from the discussion and try to explain what would be most helpful. You might find taking your questionnaires along helpful. Remember that, with chronic pain, you are your own pain manager, so be confident about the questions you have and be prepared to do your own research if necessary.

Maximising Your Control

There is no panacea for pain, no pain centre to remove, no single solution to make things better. Pain varies as much as we do. Managing your pain without using heavy-duty drugs (which gradually lose their effect anyway) has been shown consistently to involve three things:

1. **Information about the condition, knowledge about pain and the nervous systems, and the ability to act on that knowledge.** Later chapters will cover, for example, emotional well-being, pain control, planning, respite from bad pain, and tools to help you cope – but as you work through these, think about everything you've learned in this book up to this point, what you'd like to go back to, and how you can plug any gaps in your knowledge.

2. **Increasing activity and involvement with others.** Exercise and social contact have a strange role to play in pain management. Sure, they help to improve the health of your muscles, joints, circulation and respiratory system. But they also change the way your brain works, re-establishing fine connections and pathways damaged by fear of pain, stress and uncertainty. Taking control and self-managing pain will involve thinking about your current lifestyle, reflecting on feelings and relationships (your psychological well-being), and planning how to maintain your energy, using respite, aids and even the supply of homemade drugs which your body makes for you (serotonin and endorphins, or morphine-like 'happy hormones').

3. **Easing acute pain.** Getting appropriate short-term drug therapy if necessary, to ease immediate acute pain and finding longer-term, drug-free approaches to deal with chronic pain.

Key Steps for Developing Your Plan

The experience of large charities supporting people with long-term illnesses (such as arthritis, diabetes, Parkinson's and cancer) shows that self-management is fundamental for day-to-day control of chronic pain. Those with a strong sense of purpose and clear understanding of what needs to be done (that is, your plan) prosper.

Many people with chronic pain have found adopting the following approach helpful:

- Being organised, proactive, positive, independent and open to things you haven't tried before will determine how successful you will be.
- Taking charge of your medical treatment by keeping track of symptoms, pain levels, medications and possible side effects will enable you to work with your doctor to determine what works best for you.
- It's important not to allow fatigue, which accompanies pain, to become overwhelming. It is a common problem that can be caused by the underlying disease process or the stress of living day to day with the pain and limitations of a chronic disease. Psychological well-being, stress management and CBT/mindfulness, as well as using natural therapies, can help. Sleep is important to maintain your resilience and avoid slipping into a low mood.
- Even though it might seem like the last thing you want to do when you're in pain, exercise is generally beneficial for your overall health. It can strengthen muscles that

support painful joints, preserve and increase mobility, improve sleep quality, and boost your mood and sense of well-being. A pain management programme should include activities and exercise that both strengthen and relax muscles.

- Using pain-friendly tools is important – anything from walking sticks or cushioned shoes to large handled can openers – depending on the types of pain you experience.

- Healthy eating is also important in providing the body with energy to combat fatigue and in maintaining a proper weight. Eat a healthy balanced diet, adding foods with anti-inflammatory properties that are rich in antioxidants if you suffer from arthritic conditions (see pages 184–5).

- Lighten your schedule and obligations, and ask for help when you need to. Pace yourself throughout your day and take breaks to conserve energy.

- Understanding and identifying ways to overcome the anger, fear or depression that can aggravate pain can be an important part of a pain management pro-gramme. Mindfulness, avoiding rumination, and using cognitive therapy to avoid negative automatic thinking and improve psychological well-being can all help.

- A key component of psychological well-being is doing things that engage you, give you a sense of purpose and, ideally, are of value or benefit to others. Having a clear sense of your own purpose and what will help you to achieve it develops your own mental health. And this is amplified by sharing it with other people, having friends outside your home and engaging with them regularly.

- Set a specific plan for reviewing your progress on a regular basis. And take each day as it comes. You will have good days and bad days. Be flexible and keep to your plan as much as possible.

Using a Pain Diary

When I tried to improve my own pain control some years ago, a diary was strongly recommended. It showed when and how my pain came on, where I was, with whom, what I was doing, what I ate, how I slept and so on. It gave me a chance to correlate my pain with my lifestyle, activity, diet, therapies and frame of mind. The Pain Diary template shown opposite helped me to think about what I needed to address. It is a simple and easily adaptable format but you could design something for yourself if you prefer. The important thing is to keep the diary and do it consistently.

You can add columns for particular foods, the weather, your mood, the activity you were engaged in, or whatever variables you think might make a difference.

Planning Your Approach

The Pain Management Wheel shown on page 125, along with the questionnaires from the book and any ideas they

Pain Diary/Template

Date & time	Pain score	Where pain is and how it feels (acute, sharp, throbbing, shooting, etc.)	What I was doing when it began	Name, time and amount of medicine taken	Non-drug techniques I tried	How long the pain lasted	Other notes
29/3/2006 7.30am	8	Sharp pains in left hip and lower back, taking my breath away	Going from bed to shower	None	Took a warm bath instead and did gentle stretching	1½ hours	Pain reduced to 3, increased to 5 during stretching, then down to 2 within 15 minutes

have prompted, will help you to decide what your pain management approach needs to address and how urgently you need to work on it. Each aspect of pain management is identified in the circle, showing as different segments in a wheel. All the sections are important because, overall, the wheel can affect the thinking we described in Chapter 4 – increasing your sense of security and control and decreasing focus on risk and anxiety. The diagram also shows a wide variety of things you can do to help yourself.

Completing the Pain Management Wheel

To help you begin thinking about your own plan, look at each segment of the circle in turn, starting at the top with 'Understand my medical condition'. You mark a cross in the relevant shaded area: a cross in the dark grey area suggests you are well informed, understand how and why your condition has been developing and are informed about options and new approaches. If you have never tried to find out more about the condition, relying instead upon what the doctor has prescribed, you might need a cross nearer the light grey area. If you've made some efforts, place a cross in the white area.

Now move on around the wheel, assessing how well managed each aspect of your life and condition is currently and where you think some effort might pay off for you.

Some of the areas of the wheel are designed to make you think quite hard before you can judge how well you are managing currently. There is more information about them in the following chapters. Remember, as you go around the wheel, that each section represents an important factor in how much you will experience pain and how much you can reduce or make it manageable.

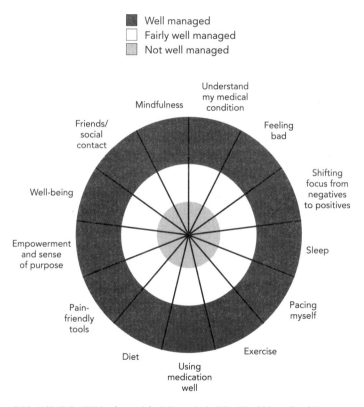

■ Well managed
□ Fairly well managed
▨ Not well managed

© Adapted by Dr David Walton from work funded in part by the Robert Wood Johnson Foundation, Richard Wanlass, Ph.D. and Debra Fishman, Psy.D., Department of Physical Medicine & Rehabilitation, UC Davis Medical Center

The first segment of the Pain Management Wheel asks, 'Do I really understand my medical condition?'

This segment asks you to think at two levels:

First, how much do you know about the medical issues you face?

(e.g. How is arthritis caused? What are the types and range of symptoms? What have other people done to cope with its effects? How does exercise help or hinder? How might the condition develop? What major risks do I face?)

Second, what do you know about your own personal condition?

(e.g. severity, likelihood of change, physical and psychological effects, recommended activity, aims of medication, timescales, risks)

Marking your cross:

Your cross should show both your understanding of the topic (in this case, your medical condition) and how you use that understanding to manage your pain.

For example, if you have suffered from arthritis for years, you might resort to painkillers first thing in the morning. Knowing more about your condition would tell you that stiffness and discomfort after sleeping are normal; many people use warm baths and gentle exercise upon waking, which helps general mobility and reduces pain levels over time. It stops you thinking that painkillers (palliatives which don't cure and can be harmful) are the only solution.

Personal (Pain Management) Improvement Goals

You could probably write an entire list of areas you might like to improve, but first you need to decide what is most important to you and not be too ambitious. Perhaps just being able to get a full night's sleep will be your starting point, eventually progressing to having enough energy to walk around a park. Once you get your pain under more control, you could consider adding other goals like getting out more, playing the piano, doing some gardening, joining an evening class or group, or swimming a few laps of the pool.

Progress may be slow and original goals may have to be adjusted from time to time to ones that are more realistic and attainable. That is to be expected and is perfectly okay. The main point is that you want to challenge yourself to improve and grow. Perhaps improvement for you is simply tying your own shoes or, on a day when you are feeling good, maybe it is walking in those shoes around the shops.

SMART goals are the most effective goals, and are most likely to help make your improvement plan a success. They are smart because they are written in a way that helps you to act and make your goals a reality. SMART goals are:

- **S**pecific: each goal must describe a specific action or step, like 'Walk to the shop' instead of 'Take a walk.'
- **M**easurable: each goal must have a specific way to evaluate it, so that you know when it has been reached, like 'Take twenty minutes to get there.'
- **A**ttainable: each goal must have your full and complete commitment behind it, like 'Walk to the shop the next time my pain allows me to go outside.'
- **R**ealistic: each goal must be possible for you to achieve, given any restrictions or limitations you may have, like 'Today my pain is worse, so I will take 45 minutes to get there.'
- **T**angible: each goal must have a reasonable target date for when you want or hope to achieve it, like 'In three months' time, I want to go shopping in the town centre, under my own steam.'

Here are some categories you can think about while making your own list of goals:

- *Physical* goals: getting back to the exercises and physical activities you love to do, like walking, jogging, cycling or going to the gym.
- *Recreational* goals: participating in your favourite hobbies and activities, such as gardening, going to the cinema or playing a sport.

- **Recovery** goals: if you have a history of alcohol or medication dependency, staying sober and/or reducing drug consumption may be one of your goals.
- **Lifestyle** goals: improving your health and outlook by quitting a habit like smoking, or by losing weight or getting regular sleep.
- **Creative** goals: getting your mind off your pain by painting, writing, playing a musical instrument or taking up a new hobby.

6. Managing Emotions and Thinking

Breathing and Emotions

Your breathing and the tension in your body are linked, and control of breathing can control how you relax. The advantage of relaxation in the management of pain, fibromyalgia and similar conditions is that as muscles become less tense, they become easier to stretch and less painful to move. Being relaxed makes you less emotionally charged, and can also help you to sleep better and feel more refreshed.

How Breathing Affects Feelings

The way we breathe is strongly linked to the way we feel. When we are relaxed we breathe slowly, and when we are anxious we breathe more quickly. When our breathing is relaxed the levels of oxygen we take in and carbon dioxide we breathe out are in balance, which enables our body to function efficiently and doesn't cause additional physiological stress. And if we exercise, our breathing rate increases, taking in more oxygen and transporting it to the muscles. In this state, we also produce more carbon dioxide, expelling it through increased breathing. Again, the body is in balance, or 'stasis'.

By contrast, when our feelings are aroused, say in a state of anxiety, the agitation we feel increases our breathing rate. We take in more oxygen and breathe out more carbon dioxide than usual, meaning that we have too much oxygen and too little carbon dioxide in our bloodstream. This reduced concentration of carbon dioxide in the blood leads to a temporary change in the pH of the blood, called respiratory alkalosis. It can lead us to feel unpleasantly light-headed, tingly in our fingers and toes, clammy and sweaty. Our heightened anxiety searches for reasons for this: 'My pain is getting worse' or 'I'm having an attack' or 'I'm so unwell I can't do anything.' When our breathing returns to its usual rate, the levels of carbon dioxide in the blood will return to normal, and the symptoms go away.

Four-minute Deep Breathing Exercise
Breathing, especially 'diaphragm breathing', or 'abdominal (belly) breathing', is a special form of relaxation which enables you to become calm and focused – which is important when you try to control emotions. This exercise can help manage your pain symptoms through relaxation but also can help you get into the frame of mind to deal with other difficult and stressful events. Here's how to do it:

Find a comfortable position either lying down on your back or sitting in a chair. Relax your shoulders. Next, place one hand on your abdomen just above your navel and below your breastbone, and the other hand on the upper part of your chest. Close your eyes and think about what your breathing feels like. As you breathe in through your nose, you should feel your abdomen rising as if it were a balloon filling with air. There should be little movement in your upper chest area. As you breathe out, do so slowly through gently pursed lips and imagine that the balloon is deflating. Try to practise this for at least four minutes. With practice, you can use diaphragm breathing wherever you are, to help relax you.

With most pain, short rest periods during the day are advisable to avoid undue fatigue and to relieve stress. Breathing techniques need to become a habit, so try to practise the exercise which follows during rest periods. At least fifteen to twenty minutes a day at first, five days a week.

Focused Breathing for Pain Control

'Breath focusing' is another exercise which helps us to resist our natural tendency for tension if we anticipate or experience discomfort. When this happens, people tend to either hold their breath or breathe in a shallow way, creating the tension.

Begin the exercise by taking a slow, deep breath from your diaphragm. Concentrate on your breathing. Breathe in – slowly – through your nose, and hold the breath for a few seconds. Then, pursing your lips, very slowly breathe out through your mouth. As you do this, think about relaxing all your muscles. It is important to concentrate on calm continuous breathing, keeping it slow and easy for at least four minutes, a couple of times each day, but when pain feels severe, use this exercise as often as you need. It is also a great time to try the 'pain gate control' exercise we will look at in Chapter 7 (see page 167).

As well as doing breathing exercises, it's helpful to explore your emotions as part of this process, so that you can incorporate strategies to control them into your self-management plan. For instance, you can guard against becoming overwhelmed by emotions if you:

- Increase your awareness of your security, safety and the positive aspects in your life. Pain and emotional fragility are worse when you feel more at risk from hopelessness, dangers and risks. See Chapter 4 for help in rebalancing safety and risk.
- Be clear what causes emotional outbursts and make tackling it part of your plan.
- Set small goals for yourself that are manageable and enjoyable – a new recipe, a new language, a visit somewhere special, a new friend, telling people when you appreciate them? Remember to make this happen by noting in your plan when you aim to achieve these goals and how you'll measure them.
- Assertiveness is about finding the right balance between meeting your own needs and dealing politely and sensitively with other people. It is not about being pushy or

selfish. Chronic pain can make even the calmest people impatient or intolerant, sometimes resulting in what appears to be an aggressive approach. So, be assertive – question the health professionals treating you about medication or any aspect of your care – but remember that they are almost always trying to help, often in difficult circumstances. Chapter 8 contains further ideas about how to be assertive rather than aggressive.

- Check your automatic pilot (how you are thinking/behaving) through the day. Do you speak to people the way you would like to be spoken to? Are you being too hard on yourself/others?

- Living with a long-term condition can knock your self-confidence in many ways and lead to emotionally driven reactions whereby you act or say things you later regret. You may not be able to socialise as much as you used to, or you may need help with certain tasks and feel bad because it challenges your sense of independence. Perhaps you have experienced changes to your appearance and weight that affect how you see yourself and what you feel capable of doing. Pain is especially hard to deal with if you don't have an effective support network, in which friends, family or your community help you to stay positive.

The remaining topics in this chapter will help you to try to control the psychological aspect of emotions, but tackling these underlying causes may become your priority.

Constructive Thinking

Thinking constructively means developing beliefs and attitudes that help you cope with pain in a more useful way. For example, a belief that managing pain is totally the responsibility of your doctor may limit you from adopting do-it-yourself approaches that are known to help others.

 Take some time to review the following pain beliefs. For those that seem true for you, try to think of a more constructive way to think about that issue. Included are suggestions to help you get started. You can use those suggestions, or come up with your own constructive ways of thinking about the issue.

Belief 1: **My pain makes it impossible to do anything constructive or enjoyable.**

Suggested alternative: Challenge the assumption that being productive or happy is impossible with pain. Start by taking note of the activities you are still able to do. Next, for activities you previously enjoyed but don't feel able to do now, explore ways you might modify them so that participation is still possible. Make sure you notice pleasurable, satisfying or even joyful moments you've experienced since the pain condition began.

Belief 2: **It is primarily the responsibility of my doctor to relieve pain.**

Suggested alternative: Start to notice and think more about small ways you have been able to manage pain. Try to implement more of these small measures into your daily life, like resting before a task instead of afterwards, or doing breathing exercises during sharp pains. Look at your self-management plan to increase your options for pain control, emphasising your outlook of 'I am secure and safe' and focusing on the aspects of life you value and enjoy. Talk with your medical team about ways to build on your personal strategies and how to combine them with medical interventions to achieve the best outcome. Be sceptical about approaches to dealing with your pain that are solely reliant on heavy-duty painkillers or opioids.

Belief 3: It is best to avoid all painful activity so that I do not cause more injury.
Suggested alternative: Ask your doctor or physiotherapist about what exercises and activities are safe and what you should expect when you are beginning to use your body more. Once you have this knowledge, practise thinking of stiffness as a sign of progress. Use the advice to avoid thinking unnecessarily of yourself as in danger.

Belief 4: My attitudes and emotions don't affect how much I suffer from my pain.
Suggested alternative: Recognise that pain is a process influenced by attitudes and emotions. Think of examples of how your pain or your ability to cope seems to change with

stress or strong emotions. Does your pain get worse when you feel stressed?

When you notice that you are taking a negative or strongly emotional view, ask yourself, 'Is this helping me or others to feel better?' Try using the focused breathing exercise instead (page 132) or focus on something which interests you, that you enjoy or are accomplished at. This helps reduce both negative emotions and pain.

Mindfulness and Meditation

'Whatever you are doing, ask yourself, what's the state of my mind just now?'

Dalai Lama, citing verse 35 of the
'Thirty-Seven Verses on the Practice of a Bodhisattva'

Mindfulness and meditation are practical techniques used to treat chronic pain, depression, surgical recovery and other physical and mental health problems. Studies in the UK, North America and Europe show they can be *more* effective than drugs, antidepressants and many forms of therapy. In general terms, mindfulness means awareness; this poses a curious paradox for people with chronic pain as we seem to be only too 'aware' of our suffering. How can becoming more aware possibly help?

Well, mindfulness is a type of reflection which begins in a similar way to meditation, but then it becomes a more active and purposeful way of thinking. Using guided imagery and relaxation, it allows you to become a more detached observer of experiences within your body and to develop greater sensitivity to what is happening around you. This allows you to detach yourself from the emotional reaction that pain causes, reducing its impact.

Thousands of scientific papers have now demonstrated that mindfulness reduces pain, enhances mental and physical well-being, and helps people deal with the stresses and strains of daily life. Here are a few of the main findings of its benefits:

- Mindfulness can dramatically reduce pain and the emotional reaction to it. Recent trials demonstrate the average pain 'unpleasantness' levels can be reduced by 57 per cent, rising to 93 per cent when carried out by experienced mindfulness practitioners.[6]
- Clinical trials show improvement of mood and quality of life in pain conditions, such as lower back pain, in disorders such as IBS and in challenging conditions like multiple sclerosis (MS) and cancer.[7]
- Mindfulness improves working memory, creativity, attention span and reaction speeds. It also enhances mental and physical stamina and resilience.[8]
- It is a potent antidote to anxiety, stress, depression, exhaustion and irritability – people who practise mindfulness are far less likely to suffer from psychological distress.[9]

- Mindfulness-based cognitive therapy (MBCT) is now one of the preferred treatments used in pain management clinics and recommended by the National Institute for Health and Care Excellence (NICE) in the UK.[10] It has many other clinically proven benefits, for example in reducing alcohol intake and drug use, and increasing brain grey matter affecting specific functions (self-awareness, empathy, self-control and attention). It also impacts on parts of the limbic system, minimising the production of stress hormones and building areas of the brain that promote positive mood and learning.[11]

These and many other studies show that mindfulness creates real, physical changes in areas of the brain that process and regulate pain, emotion and depression. They also show how it complements other therapies, demonstrating that around 65 percent of complex patients (i.e. those who haven't responded to conventional medical treatments) are less troubled by pain after learning mindfulness. It is increasingly offered, supporting clinical pain management programmes in UK hospitals.

It isn't the case that the pain simply disappears when we practise mindfulness. Instead – remembering what we discussed earlier in the book about the pain experience being controlled by your brain – mindfulness teaches you to accept what is happening in your body and to detach yourself from the emotional reaction it causes. No longer reinforced by emotion, your pain becomes weaker; you still know it is there, but your brain prevents it from becoming your sole focus, and thus makes it easier to handle. Many people who learn about mindfulness find that the *anticipation of pain* – as well as the pain itself – diminishes. This is important because the anticipation of pain triggers increased sensitivity in the central nervous system.

 In a 2012 trial, people who had practised mindfulness for more than six months and a control group of people who were not familiar with mindfulness received unpleasant electric jolts while their brains were being scanned to record differences in their effects. The mindfulness practitioners showed reduced brain activity in the brain's limbic system and reported both a reduced pain reaction (22 per cent) and reduced anticipatory anxiety response (29 per cent) when compared to the control group. Researchers concluded that mindfulness can be a powerful tool for pain management.

Exercise: Beginning Mindfulness
• Sit down at a table in a quiet space, with a small object in front of you (like a jar of jam, a cup, spoon – anything will do). Place your hands palms down on the table; think about the stress and tension flowing out of your fingers, but don't move them. Enjoy sitting comfortably and relaxed.

- Look closely at your object for a couple of minutes without touching or moving it. Don't judge its usefulness or beauty; just think about what it looks like, its shape, colour, textures, etc. Then, remaining still, gently allow your eyes to close.

- Think about the physical sensations you are experiencing as you sit there – the feel of your hands on the table, the places where your clothes touch your body, the feeling of the chair and the pressure on your bottom.

- Take a moment or two to register what you can smell or hear. It may be the scent of air freshener or coffee from a cup in front of you; perhaps the sound of your breathing, the air entering and leaving your body. Or a clock ticking. Maybe you hear noises from somewhere outside – an aeroplane, droning in the sky far above. Or maybe you spend these moments just becoming more aware of the silence surrounding you.

- Our brains are built to both generate and cope with many thoughts which come and go all the time. Your first attempts at mindfulness exercises are almost certainly going to be plagued by unanticipated distractions. Be aware of these thoughts, but try to avoid dwelling on them. Try to visualise them floating in and out of your mind like giant bubbles, and let them just drift away.

- If you become aware of some discomfort or the nagging ache of pain, try to **imagine** the flow of information coming from the problem area up to the brain and how the brain responds. **Visualise** the emotional brain exaggerating the signals, worrying that it thinks you are in imminent danger and asking your nerves to provide every tiny piece of information, about even the most irrelevant niggles. And think about the sensible bit of your brain calming the emotions, putting a duvet over them to keep them warm.

- Now allow your mind to rest, comfortably and calmly, for a few minutes, accepting any sensations you feel or sounds you may hear; then simply allow them to drift away.

- When you are ready, open your eyes and reflect on what you have just experienced. By focusing on an object initially, then on sensations and sounds, you have given yourself a break from all the things that usually preoccupy us. By recognising and accepting what is going on in your immediate surroundings and in your body, your anxieties diminish and pain can be overtaken by the new awareness of other sensations. You have allowed the rational part of your brain to have greater impact than the automatic reactions that often govern us.

These are important aspects of mindfulness. By concentrating on everything we experience now, in this very moment, we can overcome the instinctive reaction to pain, the discomfort when our brains go into emergency mode unnecessarily. Emotionally, and in our relationships with our carers and loved ones, it can be mentally refreshing and help us to value things we don't always notice.

Cognitive Behavioural Therapy

Cognitive Behavioural Therapy (CBT) is recommended for many people whose pain is accompanied by low mood, hopelessness and depression. It is frequently used alongside other methods of pain management including medication, physical therapy, weight loss, massage or, in extreme cases, surgery. But CBT is often the one which creates lasting effects. Asking you to question automatic and negative thinking, CBT targets anticipatory anxiety in which the fear of pain becomes its trigger. CBT has been shown to create physical changes, triggering natural hormones and chemical messengers, making the body's natural pain coping response more powerful.

If you're wondering whether CBT could benefit you, it helps to understand what's involved.

- CBT encourages a *problem-solving attitude*. The worst thing about pain is the sense of learned helplessness – 'There is nothing I can do about this pain.' CBT encourages action and, as a result (almost no matter what that action is), people feel more in control.
- It provides skills for *understanding your automatic reactions* to situations and helps you choose how to manage the thoughts and feelings which may cause you problems.
- CBT has been shown to help activate neurotransmitters (signals in the brain) affecting the central nervous system and *triggering the action of inhibitory*

interneurons within the spine's pain gateways. As you saw in Chapter 4, pain gates are part of the pain control mechanisms of the autonomic nervous system.

- CBT *offers a system for coping* with situations (anger, anxiety and panic attacks, trauma, body and personality disorders) that make the severity and long-term consequences of pain much worse.

CBT can be done with a therapist, individually or with a group of people. It can also be done from a self-help book or computer program. In England and Wales, two online programs have been approved for use through the NHS. FearFighter is for people with phobias or panic attacks, and has been found useful for people with pain; Beating the Blues is for people with mild to moderate depression. If you wish to explore either of these, talk to your doctor and ask if similar programs are available.

Cognitive Pain Management Techniques

Two simple examples illustrate how our thoughts and feelings can have a physical effect on us: if you are embarrassed, you might feel hot and your face might flush red. If you think about sucking on a lemon, your mouth puckers and starts to salivate. Cognitive pain management tools aim to use this mind–body connection to give us control over pain and other symptoms associated with it. A variety of approaches are available, from autogenic training (also called Emotional Freedom Technique or tapping therapy) to hypnotherapy, mindfulness, clinical hypnosis, pain management psychotherapy and other coping strategies (such as external focus of attention, neutral imagining, visualisation and pleasant imagining, dramatised storyboarding, rhythmic cognitive activity and pain ownership).

Studies show that, in general, cognitive coping strategies can provide better alleviation of pain as compared to other treatments without drugs.

Guided Imagery

This is a technique rather like a guided daydream, where you transport yourself to another time and place. Its use of imagery makes it one of the most effective strategies for reducing pain. Here are some ways to use guided imagery:

- Recall pleasant scenes from your past. For example, try to remember every detail of a special holiday or party that made you happy. Who was there? What happened? What did you talk about?
- Fill in the details of a pleasant fantasy. How would you spend a million pounds? What would be your ideal romantic encounter? What would your ideal home or garden be like?
- Sometimes warm imagery can be especially helpful, such as thinking of yourself on a warm beach or visiting a tropical island. On the other hand, if you live somewhere that is very warm, cool imagery such as a forest or shaded path may be more relaxing.

- Another form of guided imagery, sometimes called **vivid imagery**, is to think of symbols, colours or other images to represent painful parts of your body. For example, a painful joint might be visualised as the colour red, or it might look like it has a tight band around it or even a lion biting it. Now try to change the image. Make the red fade or change it to a rainbow; imagine the band stretching and loosening until it falls off. Change the lion into a purring kitten!

Distraction

The distraction technique, also referred to as externalised attention, is especially helpful to use during short activities that you know are painful or troublesome, such as climbing stairs or doing difficult tasks. It is also useful when you are having difficulty falling asleep or returning to sleep. The idea is simple: it is difficult for the mind to focus well on more than one thing at a time; by refocusing your mind's attention on something other than pain, discomfort or worries, you diminish these symptoms. Here are some examples of distractions you might use:

- While climbing stairs, plan exactly what you will do when you get to the top; be as detailed as possible. Or you might name a different bird or flower for each step. You can even try to name a bird or flower for every letter of your name, as you proceed.

- During any painful period, think of a person's name, a bird, a food or whatever for every letter of the alphabet. If you get stuck on one letter, go on to the next. (This is also a good exercise if you have problems sleeping.)

- While cleaning, think of your room as a map of a country you know well. Try to label all the furniture as regions, states or towns, going from east to west or north to south. You could also do this by imagining maps of whole continents. If geography is not your strong suit, think of the floor as your favourite big shop and locate each department.

- When getting up from a chair or out of a car, imagine that you are in space where you are almost weightless, floating effortlessly upward. Or try counting backward from one thousand by threes, each time getting as far as you can until you are standing. Try to break your old record.

- While opening a jar, think of as many creative uses as you can for the jar – anything except as a container. Or try to remember the words of a song and imagine the story it tells taking place inside the jar.

There are, of course, a million variations as to how you can refocus your mind's attention away from the pain and onto something else. Find the ones that work best for you and have fun with them.

Psychological Well-being

The variety of experiences people have and the way situations can be dominated by different personalities, strengths, weaknesses and flaws make coping with life difficult. Even more so when also coping with chronic pain. Life can be difficult, can lead to instability and people becoming vulnerable. Many psychologists believe that people living in 'negative environments' develop habits which help them cope in the short term but which are less helpful overall. Psychological well-being is the concept they use to describe 'optimal psychological functioning' in any situation: the self-confidence, positive relations, independence and sense of purpose needed for satisfaction or happiness.

In the early 2000s, US psychologist Martin Seligman explored the idea of what contributes to a sense of well-being, including in people who live with adverse social or health problems. Inspired by Aaron Beck, the founder of CBT, he introduced a model of psychological well-being consisting of five core elements. To survive and be happy, he suggested, we must experience *positive emotions*, *engagement* or involvement with something of *meaning* or value, *positive relationships* with others and a sense of *purpose* (doing things for others gives powerful meaning), and a sense of *accomplishment*, being competent and achieving things which are important to us. His work suggested that taking the effect of chronic health problems into account, psychological well-being may not develop in everyone and can be a significant source of vulnerability for others.

Psychologists (notably including an expert on resilience and recovery, US Professor Carol Ryff) have been compiling an evidence base about well-being which has now developed into a field of study called positive psychology – founded on the belief that, despite the challenges people face, striving for meaningful and fulfilled lives, being able to cope with their situations and trying to find happiness where possible is important. The following list of habits contains a selection of ideas that suggest how, as individuals, we might develop positive psychological well-being; they are described as habits because, in difficult or stressful situations, caring for or maintaining our psychological well-being should be part of our self-management plans.

Habits for Psychological Well-being

Psychological well-being is a critical element of your pain management planning – happiness, security and positivity help to calm your nervous systems and lower anxiety. But this involves regular maintenance, finding things in your life which continue to build well-being and balance or diminish the chronic pain.

Habit 1: **Savour positive experiences**. To get the most satisfaction and happiness from everyday events you need first to notice then value the positive aspects of life – savouring is a positive counterpart to just coping. It's more than simply feeling pleasure because it asks you to pay conscious attention to what is happening – not the simple reactions many of us give when we are on our daily autopilot. Mindfulness exercises can help with this.

Habit 2: **Practise recognising the good things which people do**, deserving of gratitude. Showing appreciation to others helps you train your mind to notice and focus on what's right in life. Positive psychologist Sonja Lyubomirsky has found this a key element in the happiness needed for resilience – and pain control.

Habit 3: **Understand what you are good at and play to your strengths**. When you play to your strengths you become stronger and can realise your potential. You need to find opportunities for this – finding social or work situations which foster good relationships and trust. People with chronic pain often find themselves isolated and develop poor self-images, so it's important to work against those impulses.

Habit 4: **Find things that are important to you in your everyday life which give you a sense of purpose**. Evidence shows that altruism – helping others in some way – results in huge increases in your own well-being.

Habit 5: **The happiest people have close personal relationships and active social lives**. This involves nurturing and valuing others, and overcoming conflicts, but also being clear about what individuals need from those relationships and valuing that.

Habit 6: **Be optimistic**. Pessimism puts you on the fast track to depression and rumination while optimism protects you from it, as we saw in Chapter 4. Learning optimism is psychological self-defence.

Habit 7: **Build your resilience**. Beyond simply making people feel good, daily experiences of positive emotions counteract the narrow habitual thinking (i.e. rumination, helplessness, magnification) characteristic of pain catastrophising (see Chapter 4). Positive emotions bolster resilience to subsequent pain.

Habit 8: **Set positive goals which create a sense of purpose**. Goals and motivation give us a sense of progress and satisfaction with life.

Habit 9: **Smile and laugh whenever you can**. Research shows that seeing humour in situations, and even consciously trying to laugh, increases the extent to which we notice things and see positives in them.

Habit 10: **Recognise there are many things we do not know or understand and constantly seek greater understanding**. This might refer to ethical or spiritual matters – or simply going the extra yard or two to look up the background to a news report or event which interests you. Spiritual beliefs have been shown to equip people who hold them with greater resistance to stress, pain and adversity.

7. Controlling Pain

Be Active – Reduce the Pain

Where possible, carrying out normal activities without over-doing it is important for reducing your everyday effort and pain. Your body is designed to move, but you may need to pace yourself. As you gain control of your pain, grad-ually try more movement each day. You need to balance exercise with your energy levels, physical capability and the constraints of your condition or injury. Regular activity for short periods followed or preceded by resting is better than concentrating movement into one long session. Rest time becomes important to prevent both fatigue and stiff-ness, which might discourage further activity. Try to avoid movements that are most painful, and if your pain increases when exercising, stop and seek medical advice. Otherwise, exercise regularly, even after your pain has eased. Pace yourself and try the following tips in your day-to-day life:

- *Avoid sitting in low chairs*; it makes you bend your body, requires more effort to get up and might give you more pain.
- *Avoid carrying heavy weights, particularly if you experi-ence back pain.* Read the section on pain-friendly prod-ucts (see pages 204–8).
- *Excess weight is a significant issue if you experience chronic pain.* Losing weight can be complicated and a

long-term goal, so if you feel overweight, seek advice from your doctor or healthcare adviser.

- *Keep moving.* It used to be thought that bed rest would help you recover from a bad back, but it's now recognised that people who remain active are likely to recover more quickly. This may be difficult at first if the pain is severe, but try to move around as soon as you can and aim to do a little more each day. This can range from walking around the house to walking to the shops. You may have some discomfort, but avoid anything that causes a lot of pain.
- *There is no need to wait until you are completely pain-free before returning to work.* Going back to work will help you return to a normal pattern of activity and improve well-being and can distract you from the pain. If you do, discussing the situation beforehand with your manager or human resources department can be useful.

Body Mechanics

When your joints are in good alignment, there is less stress and pressure on them and the body is better able to absorb shock. Here are some useful pointers for using our muscles and joints more efficiently to reduce stress, pain and fatigue:

- Balance the weight of objects you are carrying, pushing or pulling (e.g. instead of one heavy bag, use two lighter bags, one for each hand).

- Instead of twisting or pushing something with your fingers, use the palms of your hands, your forearms or your elbows.
- Instead of using your arms when pushing or pulling heavy objects, lean in and use your whole body to manoeuvre them. When lifting, don't allow your back to take the strain – use the powerful muscles in your legs.
- Use a sponge instead of a dishrag to mop up tables and counters. The water can be squeezed out of the sponge more easily by putting it in the sink and pressing down with your flattened hand.
- Hold objects close to your body to reduce the load. This in turn reduces fatigue and joint stress. Objects feel heavier when held farther away from your body and lighter when held closer.
- When using spray cans or bottles, push down with the side of the hand instead of the fingertips. If that doesn't work, consider any special products designed to reduce pressure on your hands.
- Close plastic containers with your elbow.
- Spare your hands from difficult-to-open refrigerator doors or cupboards by placing a strap on the handle. To open, simply place your forearm through the strap and pull.
- Instead of holding the handles of a rolling pin, place hands flat on top and roll beneath your hands.
- When pushing up from a chair, keep your hands facing palm down.

- Use your hip to close kitchen or dresser drawers.
- Use both arms to take down or hang clothes in the closet.
- Instead of placing your fingers through the handle of a coffee cup, encircle it with both hands. Mugs are especially good for this. Try cups and glasses with different shapes and textures to find out what works best for you.
- Carry your plate back to the kitchen by 'scooping' it up with the palms of both hands.
- When carrying a briefcase, use a shoulder strap and avoid using the handles. Carry a purse on your forearm or use a shoulder bag and avoid clutching it in your hand.

General Mobility and Joint Pain

If your general mobility or coordination is limited because of pain, stiffness or fatigue in the muscular 'core' – that is, the neck, shoulders, back, and hip and leg joints – the following section will offer some brief guidance on typical problems and how they can be helped. Once again, these ideas are for general information and you should always consult your doctor for advice on your specific condition.

Neck Pain

Acute neck pain is a common problem and generally nothing to worry about. Some people wake up one morning to find their neck twisted to one side and stuck in that position; this is known as acute torticollis and is a painful condition which can include the following symptoms: spasm of neck muscles, abnormal neck movements, and an awkward position of the head and neck. Acute torticollis may be congenital or caused by bad posture, sleeping without adequate neck support, or carrying heavy unbalanced weight on one side of your body. It can take up to a week to get better, but it usually lasts only 24 to 48 hours and is rarely a sign of a more serious problem.

Sometimes neck pain is the effect of trauma (like whiplash) caused by a sudden movement of the head forward, backward or sideways. It will often get better on its own or after some simple treatment in a few weeks or months, but sometimes it can cause severe and troublesome symptoms that last a long time. Common treatments involve reducing pain by using ice or heat packs, and maintaining movement and good posture to reduce pain and speed up recovery.

Pain can also result from normal age-related 'wear and tear' on the bones and cartilage in your neck. Variously named arthritic neck, cervical osteoarthritis or cervical spondylosis, it does not always cause symptoms, although in some people, bone changes can cause neck stiffness. Nearby nerves can also be squashed, resulting in pain that radiates down the arms and creates a pins and needles sensation and numbness in the hands and legs. Most cases will improve with exercise, massage and improved posture, but the above symptoms should always be checked with your doctor to exclude more severe conditions (e.g. cervical myelopathy which can cause permanent damage to the spine).

Anxiety and stress can also sometimes cause tension in your neck muscles, which can lead to pain in your neck.

When to See Your Doctor
See your doctor if the pain or stiffness does not improve after a few days or weeks, if you cannot control the pain using ordinary painkillers, or if you are worried that your neck pain could have a more serious cause because of other symptoms. Your clinician will examine your neck and check to identify any underlying condition. They may also prescribe a stronger painkiller, if needed to cope with acute pain. If you have had neck pain or stiffness for a month or more, they may suggest a physiotherapist or more tests.

Shoulder Pain
Shoulder pain is a common problem with many different causes. Most shoulder problems will affect only a small area and are short-lived. However, it can become a long-term problem, particularly for people who already have chronic pain or whose work involves prolonged, repetitive or awkward movements. Rheumatoid pain is a more serious, chronic condition in which your body's immune system mistakenly attacks your joints and other tissues, causing pain, swelling and fatigue. Osteo-pain is degenerative joint pain caused by wear and tear, and is less likely to affect the shoulders than other joints. However, it can sometimes follow on from previous shoulder injuries.

When to See Your Doctor

There are several possible causes for shoulder problems which would suggest you need to seek your doctor's advice. These include muscle or tendon inflammation or damage, injury to bones or cartilage, or pain as a result of compensating for other types of pain (e.g. hip or knee problems).

You should seek advice if your pain is the result of an injury, is particularly bad, or there is no sign of improvement after a couple of weeks. In some cases, pain in the shoulder is caused by a problem in another area, such as the neck, that is felt in the shoulder and upper back. This is known as **referred pain**. There are many other reasons why you might be experiencing shoulder pain, which could include poor posture, rotator cuff disorders (the muscles and tendons that keep the shoulder joint stable), acromioclavicular joint disorders (pain affecting the joint at the top of the shoulder), or even broken bones like the upper arm bone (humerus) or collarbone. A correct diagnosis will ensure you receive the right treatment like physiotherapy, corticosteroid injections or (worst case) surgery.

Back/hip Pain

THINK ABOUT IT

Lower back pain, and related arthritis, has recently been highlighted as one of the most prominent causes of disability worldwide by global Burden of Disease reviews. Back pain is the largest single cause of disability in the UK population (with lower back pain alone accounting for 11 per cent of the total). Over 30 million working days were lost to these conditions in 2016, and some 9 million people sought treatment for them (ranging in age from twelve to over 70 years old). Even twenty years ago, informal care and the production losses related to it cost £10.5 billion. Reports from 2008 suggest that annual medical costs for people in the US with neck, back and hip pain amounted to $86 billion.

Backache is most common in the lower back (lumbago), although it can be felt anywhere along your spine, from your neck down to your hips. In many cases, back pain will improve in a few weeks or months, although some people experience long-term pain or pain that keeps coming back. Most hip pain has a very simple explanation, for example if you've overdone it while exercising. The pain is usually caused by strained or inflamed soft tissues such as tendons, and it often clears up within a few days.

But long-term hip and lower back pain are likely to have specific causes such as inflammatory conditions (e.g. rheumatoid arthritis), musculoskeletal pain conditions (e.g. osteoarthritis) or osteoporosis and bone fragility.

Pain caused by a problem in the hip joint can be felt in the groin, down the front of the leg and in the knee. Sometimes knee pain is the only sign of a hip problem. Hip pain can also be felt in the buttock (although pain in this area can also be caused by problems with the lower back) or on the outside of the hip.

When to See Your Doctor

Back conditions can be very significant indicators of other problems. So, you should see your doctor straight away if you have severe back pain, particularly if it is accompanied by: fever; unexplained weight loss; constant pain, even after lying down; pains in your chest; losing bladder or bowel control; numbness around your genitals, buttocks or back passage; or if problems began after a trauma, such as a car accident. These problems could be a sign of something more serious and need to be assessed as soon as possible. This may result in a variety of drug- or exercise-based treatments or being referred to a musculoskeletal clinic for further assessment. At home, how you sit, stand, lie and lift can all affect the health of your hips/back.

Try to avoid placing too much pressure on your back to ensure it stays strong and supple. Use wheeled transporters for heavy weights; ensure your posture is correct and you keep your back straight when lifting; after exercise keep warm during the cooling down period; and if your back feels strained or painful, take a hot bath and use massage oils or creams. Wherever possible, try to maintain your mobility to speed up your recovery.

Reducing Minor Joint Pain, Stiffness and Fatigue

Avoid maintaining the same joint position for prolonged periods; this will help to reduce joint stiffness and prevent permanent shortening of muscles and tightening of joints.

- **Hips and knees**: Alternate between sitting and standing positions. Although the sitting position is generally recommended to reduce stress on the lower joints and prevent fatigue, it is important to get up and stretch frequently.
- **Knees**: When sitting, change the position of your legs so that your knees are periodically stretched out. This can reduce knee stiffness and pain when you return to standing.
- **Ankles**: Flex and point your toes while watching television or talking with a friend. You don't have to wait for a specific exercise time to do your stretching exercises.
- **Hands**: Avoid sustained grasps on objects. For example, take rest breaks when you are writing or cooking. Consider alternating writing tasks with computer activities.

In addition to maintaining mobility, these are things you can do to ease pressure on your joints and strengthen the surrounding muscles and tendons:

- *Reduce excess body weight* for a major effect, reducing stress on joints and general fatigue.
- *Regular exercise, such as walking and swimming*, is an excellent way of coping with many forms of muscular or joint pain. Activities such as yoga or Pilates can improve your flexibility and strengthen your core muscles. You should consider starting some gentle exercise as soon

as your pain allows. Simple exercises can help to restore your range of movement, promote strength, ease stiffness and get your body back to normal, but start by exercising very gently and build up gradually. A local physiotherapist can provide you with simple exercises designed to stretch, strengthen and stabilise the structures that support your neck, back, arms, hips and legs.

Other Approaches

- *Changing your sleeping position* can sometimes ease pain. If you sleep on your side, draw your legs up slightly towards your chest and put a pillow between your legs. If you sleep on your back, placing pillows under your knees will help maintain the normal curve of your lower back. If your pain comes from your joints, ensure your sleepwear gives you sufficient warmth during the night. A night-time ritual, such as reading a few pages before sleep, or having a warm bath or hot drink, encourages sleep. Avoid using electronic devices during this winding down time, especially those that emit blue screen light.
- Therapies including *manipulation, mobilisation and massage*, usually carried out by chiropractors, osteopaths or physiotherapists, can be very beneficial.
- *Acupuncture* is a treatment whereby fine needles are inserted at different points in the body. It has been shown to help reduce lower back pain and more general joint, head and neck pain. Evidence outlining the

benefits of acupuncture does exist, but it is not strong evidence. As a result, acupuncture treatment for lower back pain was removed from the NICE guidelines for hospital treatment in 2016, although it is still used by local doctors, as well as the majority of pain clinics and hospices in the UK.

- There is also ambiguous evidence about the value of *transcutaneous electrical nerve stimulation* (*TENS*) – but it is both recommended and sought after by chronic pain sufferers as a useful pain reduction technique. A machine is used to deliver small electrical pulses to your back through electrodes that are attached to your skin with small sticky patches; the pulses are said to stimulate endorphin production and prevent pain signals travelling from your spine to your brain. It seems to work for some, but not others, although this may be expected because of our latest understanding about the nature of our highly personalised pain experiences.

- *Good posture* will assist you greatly in preventing and recovering from muscle and joint pain as it enables you to use your muscles and joints more efficiently. Good posture also means that the three curves of your spine – neck, middle back and lower back – are gentle and small. These gentle curves provide stability and absorb shock when you walk and move. Check your posture using the following Natural Posture Test. If you already know you cannot achieve an 'ideal' posture because of body changes or long-standing bad posture habits, still try the test below. It is designed to help you find the best posture for your body.

Natural Posture Test

This is easiest performed in a chair.

1. Sit in a chair comfortably. Your lower back should be in contact with the chair back, but keep your shoulders clear (i.e. don't lean back).
2. Slump as far forward as you can. Return to your starting position.
3. Arch your back as much as you can without experiencing pain. Return to your starting posture.
4. Now try to position yourself between your slumped and arched positions. This posture should be comfortable. If it is not, adjust your position, aiming to:
   a. Keep your head erect, if possible.
   b. Relax your shoulders, not 'shrugging' or elevating them.
   c. Keep your upper back as straight but relaxed as you can.

It is helpful, if possible, to have a friend or family member present to give you feedback on how they see your posture and to talk about the most comfortable position you found.

Triggering Pain Gates

We explored the idea of the pain or nerve gates sited in your spinal column in Chapter 4. Understanding how they work provides the basis for several ways of controlling pain, both when you fear it is coming and as you experience it.

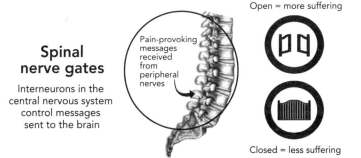

Spinal nerve gates

Interneurons in the central nervous system control messages sent to the brain

Pain-provoking messages received from peripheral nerves

Open = more suffering

Closed = less suffering

© cognitive-escape-network

First you need to know which factors open the pain gates, allowing your body to start registering pain. Pain control can start with trying to minimise how much or how frequently they open. Pain gate control involves:

- **Physical factors** (the extent of the injury or problem, too much or too little activity, the sensitivity of your nervous systems);
- **Emotional issues** (worry, tension, anxiety, anger, depression); and

- **Thinking issues** (focusing on the pain, boredom, lack of engagement, insecurity, negative perspectives and fear of risk).

If you recognise these characteristics in yourself, the projection neurons of your central nervous system will both allow and encourage greater pain sensitivity and, in turn, you will learn to anticipate pain, thus increasing pain levels.

However, this can be corrected by triggering instead 'inhibitory' neurons, which close the gates and restrict the pain signals to the brain. This happens when the brain sends neurotransmitters to 'instruct' neurons in the central nervous system to act in particular ways. The factors which encourage this are similarly:

- **Physical factors** (application of heat or ice to the injury or problem site, massage, appropriate medication and an appropriate level of activity to promote healing);
- **Emotional factors** (avoiding excessive emotions, making time to focus on positive emotions – keeping a gratitude journal, for example – and managing stress properly); and
- **Thinking issues** (visualisation of relaxation, security and calm – images of gates closing promote this – full engagement in tasks which create happiness and well-being, using a pain management plan and sticking to it carefully, increased social activities, practising positive awareness and attitudes).

There are a variety of additional actions which have also been shown to affect the closure of pain gates, including:

- Taking responsibility for your own pain management.
- Healthy (anti-inflammatory) eating.
- Minimising drug use, excluding recreational drugs altogether, avoiding smoking and controlling alcohol consumption.
- Having people around you and engaging in situations which enable you to share thoughts and feelings.

 Pain Gate Control Exercise
Record your answers to the following questions in your notebook and use it to help develop your pain management plan. The questions ask you to list some of the physical and mental factors that you are aware of when you are with or without pain. They are likely to illustrate thinking and emotional factors relevant for the pain gates to be open or closed.

What am I aware of, or what do I do, when I experience pain? (Pain gates open)

1. e.g. thinking about and dwelling on my discomfort

2. ....

3. ....

4. ....

What am I aware of, or what do I do, when I am not in pain? (Pain gates closed)

1. e.g. being with friends, planning a shopping trip

2. ....

3. ....

4. ....

Now, beginning at the top of your spine, visualise the pain gates at each of the vertebrae going down to the small of your back. Think of them as real, familiar gates you have seen or know well. Visualise the gatekeeper, the interneuron, slowly closing the gate, blocking the flow of signals designed to cause pain. Breathing deeply and exhaling slowly through pursed lips, try to visualise the flow of information from your nerves slowing down. As it does, allow the pain to drift away, fading until you can only just see it.

You can get more information about how to use pain gates either by approaching your doctor for access to a local pain clinic or by attending workshops run by clinicians specialising in pain management.

Headache and Migraine

Comedian Spike Milligan's epitaph bears this Irish inscription: *'Dúirt mé leat go raibh mé breoite'* ('I told you I was sick!'). In case anyone mistakenly thinks that this book promotes the thought that 'pain is in your head – it can't be real', let me remind you: pain is generated and experienced by the brain, but that makes it no less real. The brain is reacting to information about the body transmitted through our nervous systems, often collected from a variety of stimuli. Migraines are a good example of this complication because you feel them in your head and they are produced by the processes going on inside it. So, what's going on?

There are many types of headaches – and some of them have serious medical causes. Headaches can be a simple problem resulting from tension and stress, or they can be a symptom of something else. It is essential that you get headaches/migraines checked out, particularly if the pain is: very bad; persistent (where the pain stays very bad for a day or more or moderately bad for a week); comes on suddenly (so-called thunderclap headaches); is accompanied by a high temperature; or is accompanied by other worrying or unusual symptoms (especially weakness, disturbed vision or any neurological signs like facial muscle weakness, arm weakness or speech difficulty).

REMEMBER THIS!!!

The most common types of headaches are tension-related headaches and the more severe migraines. Almost everyone has experienced the tension headache, but research on migraines shows a more complicated picture. For example, data from the Mayo Clinic question whether sex or culture/reporting bias is responsible for 17 per cent of women in their studies reporting migraines compared to 6 per cent of men.

Migraines are sometimes described as one of the most disabling conditions because of the pain they create and the difficulty coping with it.

Tension headaches are strongly associated with stress, fatigue and neck pain, and are usually caused by nerve signals from sensitive structures in the neck, face, jaw and scalp, especially the suboccipital muscle group. Easy treatment options include relaxation, insomnia treatment, heat and ice, breathing exercises, and both general and specific exercise (especially neck strength training). Mindfulness has been found to have a significant benefit. Self-massage of facial muscles is often overlooked but can be effective. And it is always worth having an eye examination in case vision problems are causing the headaches.

Migraines are usually worse than tension headaches, although 'just' a tension headache can be fierce. Migraines may or may not be severe but have many distinctive features. In adults, they often affect one side of the head (typically in front or near the temple). An episode can last from a few hours to three days. Migraines seem to *pound* in sync with your pulse, but researchers currently believe that your heart is less involved than the brain in creating this effect. They suggest that alpha wave activity (electrical activity in the brain and cranial nerves) and neurotransmitter function (like serotonin) are very important. Light sensitivity (optic nerve sensitivity) is common and can be severe. Migraines may be caused or aggravated by physical exertion, or triggered by foods and smells, most famously wine and chocolate.

Some features of migraines (although these are not universal) include visual, auditory and other neurological disturbances. Examples could be seeing shapes, bright spots or flashes; hearing noises or music; experiencing jerking, twitching, pins and needles or even trouble speaking. These sometimes develop over five to twenty minutes and last for up to an hour, and for some people suggest that a migraine is imminent.

It's also possible to experience a variety of other migraine warning symptoms for up to two days beforehand: including fatigue, mental fog, neck stiffness, constipation and strong food cravings. *Osmophobia* is smell intolerance, and a 2007 study found that it is exclusively a migraine symptom, occurring in about 40 per cent of migraine patients, but not at all in those with tension headaches. Being particularly offended by smells during your headaches strongly suggests migraines.

The exact cause of migraines is unknown, although they're thought to be the result of temporary changes in the chemicals, nerves and blood vessels in the brain. Around half of all people who experience migraines also have a close relative with the condition, suggesting that genes may play a role. Some people find migraine attacks are associated with certain triggers, which can include hormonal changes, emotional triggers like stress, anxiety, tension, shock or over-excitement, certain foods or drinks, and major temperature change.

Treating Migraines

While there is currently no cure for migraines, a number of treatments are available to help reduce the symptoms, including:

- Painkillers – including over-the-counter medications such as paracetamol and ibuprofen
- Triptans – medications that can help reverse the changes in the brain that may cause migraines
- Anti-emetics – medications often used to reduce nausea and vomiting
- Lying in a darkened room
- Anecdotally, some people find that flat fizzy drinks, particularly colas containing aspirin or soda/seltzer drinks, can help reduce the intensity of milder migraines
- Training in relaxation techniques, mindfulness and creative visualisation.

Drugs and Over-the-counter Painkillers

No-one starts taking doctor-prescribed painkillers with the intention of becoming addicted. Typically, people start taking these medications to ease post-surgery pain or to deal with pain related to diseases, such as cancer, or chronic pain following an injury. Over-the-counter (OTC) painkillers initially work well with little effort, so most of us have dropped into a habit of using them without thinking.

Rather than exploring alternative pain management techniques, which takes some effort and may not eliminate pain in the same way as drugs, people reach for the pill bottle.

Ease of use and the effectiveness of over-the-counter painkillers may lead some to reach for the drugs more often than is safe or necessary, and addiction is always a possibility, even with over-the-counter medication. They are also a convenient way of distancing yourself from emotional and more intractable issues; drugs seem to 'make it all go away'. Over time, they are often used to manage negative emotions, and it is unsurprising that people with mood disorders or emotional trauma (from, for example, accidents or illness) are more likely to use prescription pain drugs.

Much of this may be a cultural issue: a pressurised clinician may opt for a convenient drug as the first approach; and accessing non-drug alternatives for pain management is much harder than getting painkillers, even when you might want to try them.

In the US, prescriptions of opioid drugs (see below) quadrupled between 1999 and 2013, and other countries have followed similar trajectories. The number of deaths from overdoses rose by exactly the same rate. Perhaps one of the reasons for this is that taking painkillers can be pleasurable, some providing a feeling of euphoria, others giving the sense of relaxation similar to that developed through yoga or meditation, but without the (minimal) effort required. Relaxation is an important side effect of these drugs, because most people tense up when they feel pain. Similarly, instead of finding other ways to resolve pain or correct bad habits (improving posture, increasing exercise), people often take more painkillers, creating a vicious cycle which obscures underlying problems. The problem is made worse by the need for ever increasing doses because of the tolerances people build up over time.

But the risks associated with using drugs for pain management need to be balanced with their value. Many people with pain have other conditions which need to be treated. So, they are often prescribed either pain-relieving or disease-controlling medication (or both). There are vast numbers of drugs, doing very different things. As part of your self-management plan you are being encouraged to really understand what is causing your pain; that extends to understanding the drugs you are being given and what they do.

- Make sure you are absolutely clear about why you need to take the medication.

- Understand dosages, how much of each drug you should be taking, how often and when.
- Be sure to check whether they are best after meals or on an empty stomach.
- Check how quickly the drug is likely to act and how you will know when it does.
- Read the leaflets about side effects and know what to do if they occur.

To help you with managing your decisions about and use of painkilling drugs, the following sections provide some information about drugs which you may encounter. If you need to know more, ask your doctor for advice or seek it independently through pharmacists, medical standards organisations or patient groups for your particular condition. Information is available through the internet on these matters, but medical advice on it can be varied and inconsistent. Your best source will be the doctor treating you.

Painkillers (Analgesics)

An analgesic is simply a drug which controls pain; there are many different types, working in different ways. They have varying strengths, as shown in the examples below:

- *Non-opioid painkillers*, such as paracetamol, are least strong
- *Mild opioids*, such as codeine, are more potent
- *Strong opioids*, such as morphine, are the most powerful.

An **opioid** is a chemical that works by binding to special opioid receptors in the body (found mostly in the central nervous system and gut), which reduces the pain we feel. You should never exceed the recommended dose of any painkiller, but the level of prescribing currently is so great that misuse of these drugs is widespread. People with chronic pain can take some simple action to reduce their risk of opioid dependence. These include:

- Read, then follow closely, the directions on the label for prescription medication or the leaflet produced by the manufacturer.
- Be aware of potential interactions with alcohol and other drugs.
- Be alert to your risk of low mood or emotional problems because these can encourage overuse.
- Never use medication from another person's prescription, and never share your prescription medication with others.
- Never stop or change the dosage without consulting your physician.
- Safely store prescription stimulants, sedatives and opioids in a locked or childproof cabinet.

Codeine, the crucial ingredient in extra-strength painkillers, is also a member of the opiate family of drugs. Codeine induces a feeling of calm and well-being – but if taken in big enough doses, for some people it can be addictive, with significant side effects if they try to stop. Medication abuse is a widespread problem and even OTC painkillers, if abused, can be the cause of severe headaches, digestive system problems and back pain. Both ibuprofen and paracetamol, if taken beyond the recommended safe dose, can cause serious and life-threatening illnesses. With codeine products, people become hooked on the feeling of well-being, but of course, as with heroin, eventually you need it just to feel normal.

REMEMBER THIS!!! Painkilling tablets, capsules and gels also *combine* ingredients such as the analgesic itself (paracetamol) along with, for example, caffeine and aspirin. In certain circumstances this combination can cause problems; they may deal with your pain but they may also exacerbate other and perhaps even unrelated conditions.

Aspirin, for example, relieves pain and reduces the risk of serious problems such as heart attacks and strokes. But if you have had an allergic reaction in the past to non-steroidal anti-inflammatory drugs (see NSAIDs, below), such as ibuprofen, or if you have asthma, ulcers, liver or kidney problems, haemophilia or uncontrolled high blood pressure, you need to take medical advice before taking the aspirin. So, read the labels and take seriously the advice they give.

Even combined analgesics come in varying strengths, whether bought over the counter or by prescription. If you have doubts or concerns, talk to your pharmacist or doctor. Paracetamol is the simplest, safest painkiller and the best one to try first.

Non-Steroidal Anti-Inflammatory Drugs (NSAIDs)

There are many NSAIDs – aspirin, ibuprofen, diclofenac and naproxen among the most common. They act to reduce inflammation and swelling and the pain they cause.

While many people have no problems with them, they come with warnings – digestive upset, diarrhoea or stomach bleeding being the most common. You may need an anti-ulcer pill (known as proton pump inhibitors) at the same time. If used at higher doses for prolonged periods, older NSAIDs and (the newer, safer) Cox-2 inhibitors can cause blood pressure or heart problems. If you also have an illness controlled with disease-modifying drugs (see next page), you may not need NSAIDs.

Nerve Pain Drugs

Nerve pain can be severe and unpleasant, and drugs such as amitriptyline are often a first treatment. Medicines used to treat chronic neuropathic pain (NeP) often lose their effectiveness over time, however, and some only work for a small proportion of people. You may not benefit from the first drug tried, so your doctor may need to try more than one to tackle symptoms. UK guidelines say drugs such as gabapentin and pregabalin may be over-prescribed for NeP, and current evidence suggests that the risk of misuse may be greater with pregabalin than gabapentin. Patients are unlikely to develop a response after four weeks. Regular reassessment by your doctor and stopping medication that is not working effectively are important. For those required to stop medication, NeP patients attending pain clinics say they benefited from gentle physical exercise instead.

Disease-modifying Drugs

Immunosuppressive drugs help to dampen down the immune system's attack on joints in diseases like rheumatoid arthritis, fibromyalgia or lupus. Other types of drugs (known as biologics) reduce pain and inflammation by suppressing the action of certain proteins (in the tumour necrosis factor superfamily, TNF). Their use is governed by strict guidelines in assessing anyone for treatment. Not everyone is suitable, but they can offer real help for some people with rheumatoid arthritis, ankylosing spondylitis or psoriatic arthritis who haven't been helped by other disease-modifying drugs.

Steroids

Sometimes called corticosteroids, they are very powerful and can help reduce inflammation. In tablet or injection forms, your doctor will always aim for the lowest possible dose, to guard against potentially serious side effects including weight gain, high blood pressure, osteoporosis or diabetes. A key point if you are prescribed a dose of steroids – don't stop taking them suddenly. This can be dangerous. So, if you want to stop, talk to your doctor first.

Antidepressants

Your doctor may prescribe small doses of antidepressant to help break the cycle of pain and stress. They can improve tolerance to pain and, if taken shortly before bedtime, can improve sleep quality.

The brain releases a neurotransmitter called serotonin, which plays a significant part in the body's pain control process and helps to stabilise low mood too. Selective serotonin re-uptake inhibitors (SSRIs) rebalance the depletion of serotonin; depletion accompanies and is accelerated by the cognitive changes brought on by depression and low mood. SSRIs are sometimes used in conjunction with other pain modification techniques like CBT and mindfulness.

In some situations, a doctor may also prescribe tranquillisers to reduce muscle tension and painful muscular spasms.

Tranquillisers

Benzodiazepines are prescription medicines, sometimes used for short-term treatment of anxiety, sleeping problems, epilepsy and other disorders. Examples include diazepam, temazepam and clonazepam. Hypnotic and sedative medications work, in general, by increasing the activity of gamma-aminobutyric acid (GABA), a neurotransmitter in the brain. GABA is also found in certain foods like almonds, brown rice and oats. Increases in GABA activity in the brain produce drowsiness and facilitate or maintain sleep.

Research shows that four in every ten people who take tranquillisers daily for more than six weeks become addicted. Side effects can include loss of balance, cognitive impairment, dependence and an increased risk of dementia. Stopping tranquillisers can produce difficult withdrawal symptoms. Recent data also suggest a similar safety concern with melatonin, sometimes prescribed for older people with sleeping problems.

Expectancy Effect of New Drugs

The 'placebo' effect, or 'expectancy' effect, refers to people noticing an improvement in their condition not because of the efficacy of a particular drug or treatment, but because they *expected* it to work. Placebo pills are often used with control groups in testing real medicines to determine whether any positive effects are the result of the drug being tested or of patient belief.

In one study of this effect, patients with fibromyalgia were told that a new drug was intended to reduce pain. They concluded that it was effective, for several hours. The 'drug' was simply a caffeine tablet about the strength of a cup of coffee. Caffeine can improve the effectiveness of over-the-counter pain-relieving drugs, but only by a very small margin. The reduction of pain the patients experienced then was a result of their expectations of the drug, not its constituents.

When chronic pain patients are prescribed new drugs, a temporary expectancy effect comes into play. It can last two to three weeks, during which it may have an 'expected effect', so more time is needed to assess the drug's real effectiveness. Before taking any new drug for the first time, a review period (perhaps six to eight weeks) should be agreed so you can establish how well it is working for you.

REMEMBER THIS!!! Your pain management plan gives you the opportunity to consider a variety of ways to begin managing your pain, and there are more ideas in this chapter. The treatment plan which your doctor will have established for you may contain the use of drugs, and you should continue to use them. However, it is important to be realistic as to their benefits.

Many clinical trials for pain drugs target 50 per cent improvement as a goal. It is unrealistic to expect complete removal of all pain (a 100 per cent reduction). You may need to complement drugs with other forms of pain control. And, because our tolerance builds over time, you may have a choice of continually swapping drugs to find those that work, or in the long term developing your ability to self-manage your pain. Now is a good time to start doing that.

So, if your doctor prescribes a new drug, always ask what effect it should have, over what period. It is also essential to know the common side effects and when the drug's effectiveness will be reviewed.

Over-the-counter Painkillers

Lying awake, staring into the darkness, 39-year-old computer consultant Mark Edwards tried desperately to relax and go back to sleep. As his wife Julie slept beside him, Mark fought to ignore the dull ache that was beginning to creep into his joints, and the pounding headache that was adding to his insomnia.

Finally, he could bear it no longer. Getting quietly out of bed, he went downstairs to rummage in his work briefcase. There he found what he was looking for – different branded packets of strong ibuprofen and codeine. Taking some of each for the third time that night, he gulped down six tablets in one go.

Back in bed, he waited for the familiar feeling of calm and contentment to wash over him, and within fifteen minutes was sound asleep.

That night, like so many other nights before, Mark had taken 24 tablets over an eight-hour period. He was getting through 30 tablets a day – five times the recommended safe limit.

Mark was in the grip of a 'silent addiction' to over-the-counter painkillers. It can be more insidious, harder to pinpoint and easier to ignore than other drug addictions. In 2015, it is estimated that 950,000 people in the UK were misusing branded OTC painkillers containing codeine. Like thousands of other people, Mark was abusing the painkillers – it was an addiction.

Unwittingly, he was putting himself at risk of liver failure, serious stomach damage, gall bladder problems, irritable bowel syndrome and respiratory problems – yet he had no idea he was an addict.

Then, in 2003, the management team changed at work, Mark began to feel stressed, and his tablet intake escalated. When he faced up to the fact that he had a problem and tried to give the painkillers up, he suffered terrible physical and psychological side effects almost immediately, and so resumed the habit. A year later, suffering from a bad chest infection, he visited his doctor who discovered that his blood pressure was through the roof. After testing his liver function, she put him on an antidepressant to help him cope with painkiller withdrawal. It took nine months on the antidepressant for him to overcome the addiction.

Food, Pain and the 'Inflammatory' Response

Inflammation is part of the body's immune response; without it, we can't heal. But when it's out of control – as in rheumatoid arthritis or an overexcited nervous system producing chronic pain – it can damage both the brain and body, and play a part in progressing several painful conditions.[12]

But as far as self-management of pain is concerned, can foods help to keep excessive inflammation under control? While there is no specific diet that people with chronic pain should follow, researchers have identified certain foods that can help control inflammation. Many of them are found in the so-called Mediterranean diet, which emphasises fish, vegetables and olive oil, among other staples.[13]

Complementary and Alternative Medicines (CAMs)

These are treatments that fall outside of mainstream healthcare, and many doctors consider inconsistency of effect and lack of evidence for their benefits a major problem. However, there is a wealth of anecdotal evidence that some people find some treatments valuable, and their use in a limited number of circumstances has been recommended by clinicians: for example, the Alexander technique for Parkinson's disease, herbal ginger and acupressure for reducing sickness, massage and manipulative therapies for lower back pain.

Western medicine is largely evidence based, so the lack of evidence about consistency and effectiveness must be taken seriously. However, as we have seen, pain responses are highly individual; the cognitive and emotional factors influencing them are important. When complementary therapies help people to relax, trigger new ways of thinking and focus on hope rather than risk, it may be much more than a placebo effect; the neurological processes (described in Chapter 3) which affect oversensitivity in our nervous systems could be the physical mechanism by which pain is alleviated. So, techniques like mindfulness, meditation, yoga, hypnotism and aromatherapy are increasingly becoming part of mainstream medicine.

However, if you are thinking of using CAM for severe

pain relief, **first see your doctor. Don't visit a CAM practitioner instead of seeing your clinician**. It's particularly important if you have a pre-existing health condition or are pregnant. Some CAM treatments may interact with medicines that you are taking.

There is no universally agreed definition of CAMs. Although 'complementary and alternative' is often used as a single category, it can be useful to distinguish between the two terms. When a non-mainstream practice is used *together with* conventional medicine, it's considered '*complementary*'. When a non-mainstream practice is used *instead of* conventional medicine, it's considered '*alternative*', and these are usually only seen to be of value if there are no other treatments available.

 The most common complementary and alternative treatments include:

- homeopathy
- acupuncture
- osteopathy
- chiropractic care
- herbal medicines
- aromatherapy
- hydrotherapy
- tapping therapy
- reflexology
- healing crystals

- colonic irrigation
- yoga
- meditation
- cranial stimulation
- Ayurvedic medicine
- Bowen therapy
- hypnotherapy
- massage
- reiki

Deciding Whether to Use Complementary or Alternative Treatments

Generally, complementary and alternative therapies are relatively safe, although there are some risks associated with specific therapies (e.g. deep massage). In some cases, risks are more to do with the therapist than the therapy, so it's important to go to a legally registered therapist or one who has a published code of ethics and is fully insured. If you decide to try therapies or supplements, you should be critical of what they're doing for you, and base your decision to continue on whether there is any tangible improvement for your condition.

Questions to ask before beginning treatment with a CAM therapist:

- What type of qualifications does the practitioner hold and are those qualifications nationally recognised?
- What treatments are available and how long will the treatment last?
- Are there any people who should not use this treatment?
- What side effects might the treatment cause?
- Is there anything I should do to prepare for treatment?
- How much will the treatment cost?
- What system does the practitioner have for dealing with complaints about their treatment or service?
- Can they provide documentary proof that they are a member of their professional association or voluntary register?

- Can they provide documentary proof that they are insured for any damage which may happen?
- Can they provide written references from others they have treated?

You can find out more about CAM therapies either by researching them on the internet or more usefully by talking to people who have used them. The following therapies are examples of those used by people with chronic pain who have attended recent pain clinics.

Acupuncture

Acupuncture has been a mainstay of medical treatment in certain parts of the world for 4,000 years, and recent studies have begun to show the physical mechanisms by which it works. Adenosine – a natural painkiller – is a molecule in our bodies which may control how acupuncture relieves pain. Adenosine is known to have many roles in the body, including regulating sleep and reducing inflammation; it becomes active in the skin after an injury, acting as a local painkiller. Research has found accumulations of these molecules in tissues surrounding acupuncture sites. In one test, during and immediately after an acupuncture treatment, the level of adenosine in the tissues near the needles was found to be 24 times greater than before the treatment; using a drug which extends the effects of adenosine, researchers found that the benefits of acupuncture lasted three times as long.

Chronic pain patients in recent clinics have successfully used acupuncture for lower back pain and described both the treatments and particularly the discussions with therapists beforehand as beneficial. They found that the experience was calming and provided valuable information about the treatment. While therapists often described 'meridians and energy pathways', medical researchers have pointed out that acupuncture may mediate its effects in a number of different ways. The British Pain Society states: 'We have known for a long time that acupuncture alters the response to pain by modulation of some of the pain pathways in the spinal cord, and by the release of endorphins. It is very interesting that scientists have found an alteration in the tissue levels of adenosine, which helps to explain some of the modulatory effects of acupuncture on pain perception.'

Your doctor will be able to put you in touch with a qualified practitioner.

Herbalism

Medicine drawn from herbs and other plants, the origins of herbalism go back millennia; but modern-day medical herbalists make use of plants whose traditional uses are backed up by scientific research and clinical trials. However, most herbs have not been *completely* tested for effectiveness or to measure their interaction with other herbs, supplements, medicines or foods. It is important to understand that 'natural' does not mean 'safe'. This was a major issue in two recent pain clinics where chronic pain patients were convinced that herbal medicines were completely safe.

In reality, taking a herbal medicine for pain relief may not be suitable for:

- People taking other medicines
- People with serious health conditions, such as liver or kidney disease
- People who have had or are planning to have surgery
- Pregnant or breastfeeding women
- The elderly
- Children – as with all medicines, herbal medicines should be kept out of the sight and reach of children.

Once again, it is important to discuss any plans for taking herbal medicines with your doctor or qualified pharmacist.

Reflexology

Before exploring pain mechanisms and self-management, a small number (eight) of my recent pain clinic participants decided to try *alternative* (rather than complementary) therapies, beginning with reflexology. Pressure is applied to zones of the body (usually hands and feet) in the belief that the area chosen will create physical change in another area or organ. There is little consistent medical evidence for reflexology's effectiveness but, surprisingly, half of those trying reflexology did find their pain receded. The effect was temporary, however, lasting hours rather than days. The group subsequently decided that the benefit may have been related to the relaxation and calming effect that everyone reported, rather than the therapy itself.

Osteopathy/Chiropractic/Massage Therapies

Osteopaths and chiropractors are regulated professions offering, in general, massage and physical manipulation of the muscles, bones or joints to diagnose and then resolve pain-related musculoskeletal problems.

A chiropractor uses spinal manipulation – using their hands to apply force to the muscles, bones and joints in and around the spine with short sharp movements – to gradually move your joints into better alignment. They believe this relieves trapped nerves or any related problems which compromise the nervous systems. They mainly focus on muscle or joint pain.

Most people who see an osteopath do so for help with a broader range of conditions than a chiropractor would normally work with: conditions like sports and work injuries, arthritis, lower back pain, neck and shoulder pain, elbow conditions like tennis elbow, and problems with the pelvis, hips and legs. The osteopath will use physical manipulation, stretching and massage to increase joint mobility and relax muscles and soft tissues, enhancing the blood supply to damaged tissues to promote healing. They often spend more time talking to patients to diagnose health problems and are more likely to refer people to hospital for further tests.

Massage and muscle/joint manipulation are also important tools for physiotherapists, a regulated clinical profession using movement and exercise to help improve your mobility and function. They look at the whole body, rather than focusing on the individual factors of an injury; following surgery or accidents, physiotherapists use a wide variety of exercises, including swimming, which target the way the body's joints and muscles form an interconnected structure. Designed to improve movement and strength, these can be very beneficial for toning muscles, improving blood flow and providing relief from localised pain.

Pain clinic participants attending each of these therapies reported minor short-term improvements in pain (and pain actually increased for some following visits for chiropractic treatment). However, the therapists frequently suggested lifestyle changes and self-management which they found beneficial in the long term.

Hydrotherapy

Usually overseen by a physiotherapist, hydrotherapy allows you to exercise painful areas in a soothing warm water pool. The temperature encourages a sense of well-being, muscle relaxation and easing of muscular or skeletal pain. Water is weight bearing, enabling you to increase your range of movement, and allowing pain to decrease. Some hospitals have hydrotherapy pools; in other areas, physiotherapists book time in local pools solely for hydrotherapy classes.

Clinical Hypnosis

Hypnosis is a complex phenomenon with simple outcomes. When people are in a 'day-dreaming' hypnotised state, therapists working with them may be able to: help control their pain; remove the pre- and postoperative anxiety that causes pain; decrease inflammatory pain responses by cooling sensitive tissues following trauma; relieve muscle spasms causing or caused by pain; or reduce emotional factors associated with chronic pain conditions.

Different perspectives on why and how hypnosis works have emerged: according to physiologist Ivan Pavlov, hypnosis is a form of sleep or conditioned response. Psychoanalyst Sándor Ferenczi thought it was a regression to childhood fear of a parent. Psychologists White, Sarbin and Barber theorised that it is rapport with a therapist which motivates people to behave 'appropriately' for the suggestions made to them. In reality, none of these is a completely workable explanation. As late as 2016, this absence of a fundamental explanation had fostered debate about the value of hypnosis, and in a German study of hypnosis evidence, researchers concluded that the evidence was simply insufficient to support the claims made for it. However, the same study acknowledged that hypnosis results were superior to other treatments with respect to the reduction of pain and emotional stress during medical interventions and the reduction of irritable bowel symptoms.

The British Medical Association (BMA) was among the first professional organisations to investigate hypnotherapy as a potential treatment for pain. As long ago as 1892, the BMA released the findings of a committee of nine doctors who had performed experiments involving hypnosis. That committee found that hypnotism 'is frequently effective in relieving pain, procuring sleep, and alleviating many functional ailments'.

But despite their endorsement, medical professionals continued to dismiss hypnosis until the mid-twentieth century. Despite the use of hypnosis in magic stage shows, clinical hypnosis was quietly becoming more commonly used by medical and psychological professionals.

In 1955, the BMA's Psychological Medicine Group convened to ask itself the same question: 'Does hypnotherapy work?' And once again, the committee findings from 1892 were confirmed. Two years later, their final paper ('The Medical Use of Hypnotism', June 1957) was published, concluding:

> 'Hypnosis can play a useful part in … medicine
> … In responsible hands, it is a safe method of
> treatment which can be combined with others.'

Although hypnosis has been controversial because of its public (theatrical) perception, many clinicians now agree it can be a powerful, effective therapeutic technique for a wide range of conditions, including pain, anxiety and mood disorders. The profession of clinical hypnotherapist has been evolving as an accepted part of healthcare. People with chronic rather than acute pain are most frequently treated.

In 2008, when fibromyalgia patients were hypnotised in an fMRI scanner, they reported much more control over their pain and greater pain reduction than control-group patients. Scanning showed changes in the cerebellum, mid-cingulate cortex, insula and the inferior parietal cortex in their brains.

Although many people think of hypnosis as a 'deep, dreamy' state, clinical hypnotists usually work with patients only in a light, relaxed, almost 'day-dreaming' state. A less well-understood view is that we frequently hypnotise ourselves, such as when we become absorbed in what we are doing, our work, or even in TV programmes, interesting talks or religious ceremonies.

But does it really work? While modern research evidence may still be needed for certainty, studies are being published regularly that suggest hypnosis may be of great value. For example, rather than giving some surgical patients a general anaesthetic, doctors at the Institut Curie in Paris have been using hypnosis regularly to help conscious patients withstand the pre- and post-operative pain of surgery.

They performed 150 cases of surgery using hypnosis instead of simple sedation on cancer patients between 2011 and 2017, finding that in 99 per cent of cases, it worked without any problems. They used a technique called 'hypno-sedation', which combines hypnosis with anti-nausea drugs and a short-acting tranquilliser to help patients into a light hypnotic state, relaxed but conscious. Ninety per cent of the surgeries were for breast cancer (mastectomies), while the remaining 10 per cent included colonoscopies and gynaecological and plastic surgery. The patients' operations lasted about 60 minutes, under hypno-sedation alone.

fMRI scans showed hypnosis affecting the brain, increasing its ability to manage sensations the body was experiencing. The Institut believes that doctors and patients working together can use hypnosis to get patients to *disassociate from the nervous systems' response to harm* – a similar perspective to the one we discussed in Chapter 3.

To find out if the services of a clinical hypnotherapist are appropriate or available in your area, contact your doctor or healthcare provider. Alternatively, you may wish to talk to someone privately. Make sure that they are fully accredited by a professional standards body:

- Choose someone with a healthcare background – such as a doctor, psychologist, *clinical* hypnotist or counsellor.
- If you have very severe pain, mental illness or a serious underlying illness (such as cancer), make sure they're trained for working with your condition.
- If you're looking for a therapist for your child, make sure they're accredited and trained to work with children and young people.

Does Swearing Help Cope with Pain?

I described earlier in the book how there is a growing body of research into the role that emotions play in pain regulation, leading to our better understanding of the brain and its application to pain management. And we have seen that people often feel worse about their pain (and sometimes misleadingly so) when the central nervous system becomes over-sensitised.

Uttering expletives when you hurt yourself is a sensible policy, according to scientists who have shown swearing can help reduce pain. Although cursing may not be acceptable to you, neuroscience is now beginning to question whether swearing in response to pain involves more than a socialised response. The way swearing achieves its physical effects is unclear, but in studies taking place between 2009 and 2011, researchers speculated that brain circuitry linked to emotion was involved. The amygdala is an important part of that circuitry, an almond-shaped group of neurons that can trigger a fight-or-flight response in which our heart rate climbs and we become less sensitive to pain.

The researchers subjected a group of undergraduate students to a 'cold pressor test' in which the students were required to put their hand in ice water for as long as they could – until the pain was too bad. The novel part of this research was that the students did this while repeating a swear word of their choice, and later (as a control) doing it again repeating a neutral word. It was found that when swearing, students felt significantly lower pain than when

.ng neutral words. They also found that the students' .eart rates rose when they swore, a fact the researchers say suggests that the amygdala was activated.

 In a joint British and US study in 2017, it was demonstrated that the act of swearing strongly (using offensive words not a part of your normal 'cussing vocabulary' – the ruder the better!) appears to have a positive effect on strength and power. Pain regulation and resilience increase as a result.

This is probably because the body's mechanism for pain modulation is closely tied to the parts of the brain that process emotions, releasing a neurotransmitter (enkephalin) which binds to the pain-transmitting neurons in the spinal cord. Another neurotransmitter (substance P) stimulates pain receptors in the body. If a person's substance P levels are elevated, their perception of pain may be greatly exaggerated. Previous research has shown that animals lacking in substance P cannot detect increasing intensities of pain. So, the enkephalin triggered by swearing inhibits the function of substance P and reduces the pain levels experienced.

These findings add to the body of evidence on how cognitive and emotional experiences link with nerve sensitivity and chemical actions that produce and inhibit pain sensation. They point to the mechanism at work which explains why people have a higher pain tolerance when emotionally stimulated. You might like to experiment with swearing to help with your own pain. A word of caution though. If you want to use this pain-lessening effect to your advantage, you need to do less casual swearing. Swearing is emotional language. But if you overuse it, it loses its emotional attachment and thus its impact.

 When you are troubled by your own pain, *think of some **really bad** swear words* – ones which you would normally never use, the worse the better.

Choose whether you should say them under your breath, or whether you can let rip and shout them out – loud and proud!

As you become aware of your pain, repeat the swear words, concentrating on what you are saying, and think about what the words mean and how bad they are. Use stronger words if your pain keeps grabbing your attention.

Some participants in pain clinics find that to amplify the power of swearing under your breath, it helps to change the way you breathe: purse your lips, breathe in through your nose and forcibly out through your lips.

There is no time limit for this – keep going for as long as it feels useful.

---

8. Making Progress with Your Plan

Learning about pain, and the problems that people face in coping with chronic pain, can give you the confidence and security required to make a success of your own self-management plan. Most people find that they need both good motivation and resilience to be successful. There are several specific topics which people with chronic pain frequently ask about – ideas either affecting pain control or tools to help with it. This chapter looks briefly at some issues of concern raised in recent pain clinics.

Goal Setting for Your Pain Management Plan

Planning and organising how you will manage your pain saves time and energy, helps reduce fatigue and creates both motivation and a sense of purpose. It can also help get things done in your general daily life too. So, *plan* what you need to do, ahead of time.

Having read the previous two chapters and considered where your 'crosses' came on the Pain Management Wheel, think through the following questions:

- What goals shall I set for my pain management: first, for the next week/month; and second, for the coming three months?

- Is my priority immediate pain relief and, if so, which of the approaches in this book do I want to try? Can I set myself specific tasks to do, starting tomorrow?
- For each of the tasks, how important are they for me and why?
- What steps are involved in doing them?
- Will I need any help or information to achieve them?
- When is the best time to do them?
- Do I need rest periods to preserve my energy?

Pacing, Time and Energy

People with pain sometimes talk about 'good days' and 'bad days' when their pain gets in the way of daily activities. Then, 'good days' double up as 'catch-up days', finishing what couldn't be done when the pain was overwhelming. If you over-do things on a catch-up day, you may have to take out several days to recover, increasing the number of 'bad days' you experience.

One of the best ways to avoid getting over-tired is to plan short but frequent rest periods throughout the day. If you can prevent fatigue, even if it means stopping in the middle of a job, your endurance over the long run will be increased. While stopping to rest might be difficult, remember that the longer you work, the more time you will need to recover. But you don't necessarily need to sit down. One way of resting muscles is to use other ones. For example, after working at your computer or sitting at your kitchen table preparing vegetables, stand up and stretch. After an extended time in one posture, like waiting for a bus, change it by bending over, shifting from one leg to the other or flexing your shoulders and neck to relieve overused joints and muscles.

Effective pacing means that *you* (rather than your pain) are in control. It sometimes helps you to accomplish even more than you may think possible.

Here are a few ideas which might help you build pacing into your pain management plan:

- **Schedule frequent rest periods throughout the day**. An example might be to rest ten minutes out of every hour, instead of working for three hours straight. Even a short break is better than none, but plan for what *you* need rather than for others' needs.
- **Alternate heavy and light work tasks** during each day; try doing some paperwork after making the beds, or bake a cake after changing the wheel on your car. In addition, plan the more difficult or lengthier tasks for days when you will have the endurance to do them.
- Sitting uses less energy than standing, but if you're at a desk all day, **moving around at regular intervals will keep you more energetic**. Your pain levels and mobility will also be worse if you get stuck in one position.
- **Make sure everyone you relate to feels working or being with you is a positive experience**, whether it's

a work group, friends or family. Life for people with chronic pain can be so much more productive and energising if you have a strong support network and others can step in if you need a break. You may also need understanding or co-operation from others if you are going to pace yourself properly. You may decide that you can't meet other people's priorities exactly when they want you to. So, building effective relationships, explaining what you are doing, how you will achieve what's asked of you and how much you need rest when it's necessary are important tasks.

- **Break up tasks into smaller parts** – take rest breaks in between tasks.
- **Work at a steady, less intense pace** within your capability, picking off the easier, quick wins first to boost your motivation.
- **Change tasks often** and exercise different parts of your body throughout the day.
- **Give yourself little 'presents' during the day** – things you like doing and are good at, taking a little time to talk with others and share news or perspectives.
- **Build your *real* priorities into your day and note them on your pain management plan** too. Avoid making everything a 'top' priority. Six 'top priorities' needing to be accomplished at the same time will make it difficult to decide how to use your precious time and energy on the most significant tasks.

Mobility Aids

Mary was feeling isolated and lonely in her home. Her fingers and wrists gave her great pain because of chronic arthritis, and she found using the telephone a real problem. She also had difficulty remembering telephone numbers. She was advised to buy a picture pad telephone – which had extra-large buttons – which she could press with her thumb, showing pictures of family members as fast-dial buttons. She now finds dialling less painful and is able to speak with her family whenever she wants. Reduced anxiety has also helped decrease her chronic pain.

There are a number of products designed to reduce joint stress, pain and fatigue by allowing you to do things with the least amount of effort. You may find some will make a significant impact on your ability to manage everyday activities and lift your mood. For information about finding these items, contact the physiotherapy (or occupational therapy) department at your local hospital or healthcare centre.

1. Wheels

Adding wheels to items, such as utility carts, tea tables or shopping bags, will enable you to push or pull items with less friction and reduce the need for lifting and carrying. Using a trolley or attaching wheels helps avoid the strain of carrying. You might also use a wheeled suitcase to take most of the strain from your arms; you can even use them to carry paperwork.

2. Long or bulky handles

Products with long handles or long attachments let you use less force to manipulate objects and so help conserve strength. Large handles can help you to maintain a secure hold when hands are painful or weak. If your fingers do not fully close or maintain your hold on objects, bulkier handles give you the option of using your palms and wrists to exert force. This also applies to a variety of other objects:

- Buy pens, tools, kitchen utensils, etc. that are made with bulky handles (about 2.5 cm in diameter).
- You can get pencil grips from office supply stores.
- A doorknob extender allows you to open the door with the palm of the hand instead of with the fingers.
- Tape a dowel or a piece of wood to a can opener and hold on to this lengthened handle when opening cans. The pressure required to operate a butterfly can opener is extreme – use an electric or wall-mounted type instead.
- Open flip-top cans with a blunt knife.
- Foam padding added to things such as a toothbrush, pen, razor, fork or comb increases the size of the handle.
- If buttons are difficult to manipulate, get Velcro sewn onto clothing. Most supermarkets sell it.

3. Lightweight objects

Lightweight versions of much household, work and travel equipment are easier to use, carry and maintain. From a pain perspective, lightweight alternatives can reduce physical stress, reducing arthritic pain and that experienced in the weightbearing parts of the body – the back, upper body, hips, arms, wrists and hands. Examples of products for which you can find lightweight alternatives include:

- Vacuum cleaners
- Kettles
- Saucepans/skillets
- Food preparation aids
- Cleaning and laundry equipment
- Shopping bags and trolleys
- Rucksacks
- Laptops and tablets
- Suitcases.

You may know of others, but if you need help, your local physiotherapist or occupational health department can help you find examples of alternative products appropriate for your needs.

Labelling items 'lightweight' is often more a marketing device than a true comparison so, before buying it, try the appliance out in a shop. Check how comfortable it is to use and where on your body most of the weight falls. Is it really the most lightweight item available or are there alternatives for you to try? Online shopping sites will usually give you product dimensions and weight, which you can compare with other similar appliances. Shops should also have that information, but you may need to ask for it – then take the time to shop around, reviewing your options and ensuring it is the most appropriate alternative for you.

4. Convenience items

To decrease the length of time and number of steps needed to complete a task (and in so doing, reduce pain, joint stress and fatigue), you might try out these products.

- Use labour-saving powered devices such as a food processor, blender, microwave, electric toothbrush, can opener, or salt and pepper mills.
- Seats which automatically rise can help hip and back pain sufferers to stand upright and begin to move, without placing effort on particularly painful parts of the body.
- Buy non-iron or permanent-press shirts, blouses, dresses and trousers.
- Use Velcro fastening shoes and extending shoe trees if you have back pain when either trying to reach your feet or in putting your shoes on.

There are a variety of other mobility aids, including stabilising crutches, walkers, cars, scooters and stair lifts which make life easier for many people. Chronic pain can be disabling for some people and they may need to consider such aids. Information about the range of options should be available at your local healthcare centre. But where the use of an aid is no longer necessary, the convenience it offers can become a liability. Exercise is important in order to avoid the risk of losing muscle tone through lack of activity, prolonging both pain and disability. Physical activity helps activate the pain gates inhibitory interneuron we discussed in Chapters 4 and 7, maintaining your pain control.

 An old adage says: 'If you don't use it, you'll lose it.' Use mobility and pain relief aids when they can help you reduce pain, maintain activity and help you exercise. But using them when you don't need to will slow your recovery and even diminish your pain control.

Sleeping

Sleep restores energy, improves resilience for managing pain and helps the body to restore itself. It is thought that sleep helps us to cope with daily pressure too, by sorting information and memories, adjusting our body's chemical and hormonal balance, and allowing us to replenish our energy levels.

Sometimes people take a brief nap during the day, but this can be very unhelpful. Most people need a good few hours each night to replenish energy levels, although the amount is often age related. When you're in pain, trying to get to sleep can seem nigh-on impossible, and the knowledge that not getting enough sleep will make the pain even worse the next day just makes it even trickier. So, what can be done to get more and better-quality sleep?

Exercise:
Gentle exercise or stretching – within the limits of whatever condition you have that causes your pain – will help tire muscles and relax your body, while the effort expended will make sleep come more easily.

Don't over-eat, particularly at bedtime:
This applies whether you're in pain or not – and avoid stimulants like caffeine and alcohol before bed. Even though alcohol may ease pain, it'll keep your body and mind active, making it more difficult to drift off.

Focus on your breathing:
The breathing exercises in Chapter 7 will relax and calm you, reducing the anticipation of pain which makes getting to sleep difficult.

Talk to your doctor about supplements:
Certain vitamins and supplements – including melatonin, vitamin D and iron – have been shown to help reset your body's sleep patterns. A balanced diet makes supplements normally unnecessary, but if you are considering using them

for severe sleep problems, talk to your doctor. Try to avoid opioids and sleeping tablets if you can. It's also important you are taking the right dosage of any prescription pain-killers as this can also interrupt sleep patterns. So always check this with your doctor too.

Naps:
Even brief periods of sleep during the day make it much harder to fall asleep when night falls. But if you have to nap during the day, keep it to twenty minutes or less. Napping in the early part of the day is better for you, and overcome an afternoon energy slump instead with a short walk, a glass of ice water or a phone call with a friend. You can reduce the need to nap by following the advice about conserving energy contained in this chapter on Pacing, Time and Energy.

Temperature:
Keep it cool. Your body needs to drop its core tempera-ture by approximately 1.2 degrees Celsius to initiate sleep. This is the reason it's always easier to fall asleep in a room that's too cold than too hot. About 18°C (64°F) is optimal for your bedroom. That's cooler than you think, and older people may need one or two degrees warmer. It's fine to wear socks if you get cold feet. But cold it must be.

Light:
Dim your lights before bed. Switch off as many lights as pos-sible in the last hour before bed so as not to interfere with

natural production of the sleep hormone melatonin, which is produced in the evening. Blackout curtains are also helpful. Tablets and phones in particular generate lots of short wavelength blue light, which reduces melatonin concentrations. In experimental research, older people have found it easier to sleep, and gained 30 minutes more sleep, by wearing inexpensive wraparound amber-lensed sunglasses for two hours before bedtime. Turn off TVs, computers and other blue-light sources an hour before you go to bed. Cover any displays you can't shut off. In the morning, get out in bright light for five to 30 minutes as soon as you get out of bed. Light tells your body to get going and resets your hormonal balance. Many people with chronic pain have found using an especially bright 'SAD' light box first thing in the morning gives better sleep and reduces pain levels throughout the day.

Avoid rumination:
Never lie awake in bed for a significant period of time (more than twenty minutes or so); rather, get out of bed and do something quiet and relaxing until the urge to sleep returns. See advice about avoiding rumination in Chapter 6.

Block your clock:
Do you glance at your clock several times a night? That can make your mind race with thoughts about your pain, lack of sleep and the day to come, which can keep you awake. Put your alarm clock in a drawer, under your bed, or turn it away from view.

Try a leg pillow for back or leg pain:
Even mild pain can disturb the deep, restful stages of sleep. Put a pillow between your legs to align your hips better and stress your lower back/legs less. If you sleep on your back, tuck a pillow under your knees to ease pain.

Manage liquids:
Don't drink anything in the last two hours before bed. If you have to get up at night, it can be hard to get back to sleep quickly. Pass altogether on the coffee or alcohol for a nightcap. Avoid caffeine after 1pm and alcohol after 5 or 6pm. As a guide, never go to bed tipsy. Alcohol is a sedative, but sedation is not sleep. Unfortunately, most people mistake one for the other. Alcohol also blocks your REM sleep, and it further fragments it with short awakenings throughout the night. You wake up feeling unrefreshed and unrestored when having had a drink in the evening.

Get relaxed:
About an hour before you try to sleep, read something calming, meditate, do a guided visualisation exercise, listen to quiet music or take a warm bath. Avoid conversation, even with your loved ones, during this time. Even ten minutes of relaxation makes a difference. Regular night-time routines help, such as having a warm bath before bed, reading for half an hour or doing some mindfulness activities like breathing exercises or putting your mind into a resting state.

To summarise, chronic sleep loss can be a major problem for pain, recovery from health problems and maintaining mental health. So, talk about your sleep problems with your doctor, distinguishing any discussions about your underlying condition from one focusing on sleep loss.

Strengthening Relationships

Seeing a loved one (or someone close to you) in severe pain is very distressing. Coping with their frustrations, sharing their limitations and constraints or the need to do things for them which you never imagined can create major difficulties for colleagues, families and friends. Sometimes people feel closer when they face problems together but, in the face of very challenging circumstances, communication can become difficult or may even break down completely.

People in pain can feel unhappy because it has generated a sense of loss in their life, missing things they used to do and feeling no longer as strong or powerful as they did before. These feelings can have many other effects – on mood, on how people express themselves, and on family or friends trying to help. So, it's important to listen carefully to both what the other person is saying and *how* they are saying it (the underlying feelings and emotions which are such an important feature of communication). As is recognising that communication is a two-way thing. Psychologists often talk about '*behaviour breeding behaviour*' – others react to you based on how they interpret your words and intentions. We get our interpretations both right and wrong all the time. So, how aware are you of any messages you may (unwittingly) send to others with whom you spend time?

Communication problems affecting relationships (between pain sufferers and those caring for them) can often be caused by the lack of control which chronic pain can lead to. Being cared for and looked after when you are in trouble is, for most people, welcome and provides security. But when others make decisions for you – even with the best of intentions – it can make it harder for you to feel in control of your situation or that you still have a useful role to play. This can make people with pain withdraw, so that they're deliberately spending less time with others or with particular individuals. Pain can also make socialising stressful when it involves the effort of going out, moving around or even concentrating for long periods.

So what rights does someone in that situation have? This is often a contentious matter when discussed in pain clinics, particularly for older people and those with limited mobility; many participants have talked about their gratitude and reliance on carers, both for physical and emotional support. But equally they report that carers can become focused on getting things done quickly, so the independence of the person being cared for can become less important. They mention the importance of being able to express their views (including saying no to things) without being made to feel guilty; that people in pain should be able to express their appreciation to others but also express their own needs; and that both carer and sufferer should be able to solve problems by listening and showing respect for each other and recognising that both need to feel valued.

The following ideas may help reinforce the bonds between carer and someone being cared for:

- Chronic pain does affect relationships, so it's important to talk about its effects on those who are close to you.
- People need to know if you appreciate something they've done for you; thank them and let them know specifically what it was that you found helpful.
- Relationships change all the time, so if problems do occur, knowing how to talk things through can help you adapt to new circumstances, make changes and cope better. Chronic pain can lead to isolation and lack of contact with previous friends – which can make talking about subjects you feel strongly about difficult.
- It can be helpful to accept that both of you should be able to say what's on your mind, to be listened to without rancour and to talk things through without trying to punish each other.
- Focusing more on what you've achieved, successes and enjoyable events is better than constantly focusing on disability or the pain itself.
- Being able to challenge your own thoughts and feelings and being concerned about the other person's feelings is a mark of success.

- And if you are communicating well, make sure you know what sort of humour you both enjoy. Laughing together is a great way to strengthen relationships.

Communicating Assertively

As we discussed in the previous section, chronic pain can create isolation which often interferes with good communication. Assertiveness is knowing what you feel and need, and making clear choices about when and how to communicate these. But it is not about being pushy or selfish. It is about finding the right balance between meeting your own needs and dealing politely and sensitively with others. It is neither passive nor aggressive. Let's look at this distinction more closely.

Passive communication is keeping your needs to yourself, or hinting and hoping others will notice and take care of them; getting upset when others don't notice; bottling up anger and other negative feelings; manipulating others through guilt, pity, 'owing you', etc.

Aggressive communication is putting your own needs first at all times; being loud, pushy and bullying; intimidating others into doing things your way; not listening to other points of view; rarely expressing positive feelings; undermining others with sarcasm, etc.

Assertive communication is checking in with yourself as to how you are feeling; giving clear messages about what you would like; speaking calmly; respecting other people's opinions while expressing your own; having a relaxed posture and facial expression; knowing your limits and non-negotiables.

Assertive communication is something many of us struggle with, but with some attention and practice, we can start doing it better and make sure we look after our relationships with carers, as well as doctors, colleagues and others in our lives. It often begins by increasing our self-awareness. People often think that people in pain are either helpless or 'self-centred'. The truth is that pain can reduce our normal sensitivity to others and make us less aware of the effect we may have. Learning to tune in to your feelings again may take a bit of practice. Trying to maintain a calm outward approach when you are upset can feel difficult at first.

It helps to have a support network in place. Close friends can help you stay aware of your approach. It may also help to write things down. Simply keeping the pain diary helps you stay in control of what you are feeling. Rating the intensity of your feelings at different times helps you see changes and patterns, instead of a sense of being always low. Being more aware of these feelings will help you to keep them in check, instead of using them against others in communication. Expand the range of words you use for each type of feeling: contented, happy, satisfied, joyful, ecstatic, pleased, animated, chuffed … Practise using the precise word to describe your mood or feeling at any given time.

Once we've reflected internally, we might start to notice areas for improving communication:

- Make a list of situations where you feel you need to improve the communication of your feelings or needs.

- Assertive communication uses clear descriptions of situations followed by statements of what you feel or need: 'That brace broke the first time I wore it and left me in real pain. I would like to know if it is the only design available.' It is important to ensure the person you are speaking with understands that the issue you are raising is important to you and talking about its effect on you lends your points greater impact.

- Deliver statements in a calm and matter-of-fact way. No need to build up a head of steam, or to be overly placatory.

- Practise assertive communication but watch out for unnecessary pleading or manipulation in your voice.

- Make a habit of thinking about what the assertive way to communicate something would be.

- Remember that assertive communication includes choosing when and with whom you wish to communicate, and how much you want to say.

- Working it out ahead of time gives you confidence that you can keep things on your own terms.

- It's especially important to be clear about situations where you need to be better at setting limits and saying no.

There are many books on assertiveness which can give you more ideas if this is something you'd like to explore further.

THINK ABOUT IT If you are trying to manage your own pain, you know how distressing it can be. If you know elderly people or children with special needs who are in pain, you will understand that communicating their distress may be extremely difficult.

We said in Chapter 6 that part of your own well-being is enhanced if you can use your insight and ability to do something worthwhile for others.

So, the last section in this chapter is about assessing older people when you suspect they may be in pain. It is designed to help you recognise when they may need help – and perhaps you might be able to offer it.

Assessing Pain in Older People

Pain in older people is mainly associated with chronic underlying health disorders (e.g. arthritis, diabetes or cardiovascular/peripheral vascular and neurological disease), conditions such as cancer, and the consequences of surgical procedures. Older people also frequently have more disorders that coexist with other conditions (**comorbidity**) and require more complicated treatment.

Clinical research has suggested that, internationally, *many older people are at increased risk of having their pain under-assessed and under-treated*. Reasons given for this include problems dealing with patients who have dementia, a condition associated with pain-causing medical conditions such as respiratory and urinary tract infections, pressure ulcers and fall-induced fractures. Unrelieved pain can become a real problem for dementia patients, made worse by their difficulty in communicating. Older people may be hampered by multiple conditions, by depression, perhaps by a reduced ability to communicate effectively, or by their own stoic values or home remedies that leave illnesses unseen until they cause real problems. People with cognitive impairment may also be unable to describe what they feel and report symptoms, which in turn complicates the diagnosis of other pain-causing comorbid conditions. Physiological and psychological distress, particularly for older people who live alone, can result in increasing disorientation and the emergence of behaviours that challenge carers and healthcare providers. There is, too, the general view that chronic pain requires much more time to understand and treat, by clinicians for whom time can be scarce.

Arguing in 2014 for better, more comprehensive treatment planning for pain in older people, the British Pain Society and Age UK drew attention to very large numbers of over 65s who are in pain or discomfort, particularly those in institutionalised care settings. The incidence of cancer pain for this group is widespread and has long been recognised as having a profound impact on their quality of life. Older people themselves have talked about pain, and you can see a few of their views in Chapter 1. Their experience, and those of others, have led to the development of standardised guidelines in the UK and elsewhere for the use of drugs and opioids in the treatment of major conditions affecting older people, and the use of psychological therapies and self-management guidelines such as those in this book. However, the challenges for improving pain assessment and self-management are complex. Once again, studies show the importance of taking time for an individualised approach to these issues.

In 2014, an American research group on 'persistent pain in older persons' outlined six areas that might help carers and clinicians to assess levels of pain when older people are unable to verbalise exactly what is happening to them. The following questionnaire, based on those areas, may help you to assess pain levels in older people whom you suspect may be in chronic pain.

Questionnaire 4:
Assessing Pain in Older People

Think about each of the areas described in these questions.
Give a score for each area, then look at your overall assessment.
It would be helpful if you then called on a clinician, describing
exactly what has given rise to your concerns.

1. **Facial expressions**. Looking tense, frightened and grimacing
   has been shown to increase during movement, especially in
   those with cognitive impairment. Several facial actions characteristic of pain have been identified, including brow raising,
   brow lowering, cheek raising, eyelids tightening, nose wrin-
   kling, lip corner pulling, chin raising, lip puckering, etc.

0	1	2	3
Absent	Mild	Moderate	Severe

2. **Negative vocalisation**. Changes can include aggression and
   withdrawal, and are particularly important to notice in cogni-
   tively impaired patients with severe communication problems
   who may be reticent or unable to report pain problems.
   Different patients have different vocalisations and pain behaviours, e.g. clutching painful areas, groaning, sighing, grunting,
   weeping or whimpering.

0	1	2	3
Absent	Mild	Moderate	Severe

3. **Body movement**. Clutching and rocking, guarding (abnor-
   mally stiff, rigid postures) and, to a lesser extent, bracing
   (maintaining a stationary position of the limbs) can be used
   to detect movement-exacerbated pain. Physiological change

is also important, including temperature change, redness or flushing, pallor and sweating.

0	1	2	3
Absent	Mild	Moderate	Severe

4. **Changes in levels of activity** or types of things they do. Generally, pain will prompt people to do less and increase the amount of sitting, lying or manoeuvring they do. There are significant problems which stem from this: the tendency to avoid movement and exercise can make many conditions (such as arthritis) worse, and 'self-labelling' as ill enhances catastrophising (described in Chapter 6).

0	1	2	3
Absent	Mild	Moderate	Severe

5. **Changes in interpersonal interactions**, such as refusing to eat, an increase in confusion, withdrawal from interacting, greater volatility and other alterations to interactions with normal contacts.

0	1	2	3
Absent	Mild	Moderate	Severe

6. **Mental status changes**. Greater memory problems, confusion and the ability to use information may be a matter of degree for those with an existing dementia diagnosis; older people may have various patterns of talking, thinking or working out problems – any changes to these may help with understanding the levels of discomfort felt.

0	1	2	3
Absent	Mild	Moderate	Severe

Total _____

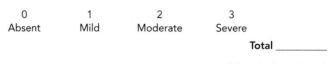

Final Thoughts
– Now the Journey Begins ...

So, now is the time to review your notes and thinking and to work out your goals, targets and priorities for your personal pain management plan. As we said at the beginning of the book, when you understand how chronic pain works, and understand that there are physiological explanations for the way thinking affects pain intensity, a whole new set of possibilities open for you to control and manage it.

There is a growing recognition that if you have chronic pain, you will benefit greatly from taking charge of pain control, getting help from clinicians and friends – but taking responsibility for how you control it personally. People with similar conditions and pain level differ in their response to pain management, so it is vital that you make a plan which works for you – whatever you decide to include. There is strong evidence that developing your own plan will not only help you to control your pain better, but it may also reduce frustration, depression and other mood disorders which frequently follow chronic pain.

Remember that your control will be more effective when you understand what your condition is, the risks (if any), and the fact that pain is only part of your life. Remember that valuing all the other, good, things – the things which keep you safe and secure – and keeping them constantly in your focus will help enormously. Not by magic though. Doing this helps to rebalance an overexcited set of nervous systems and makes pain control more effective.

Hopefully the key principles on which the book is based will help you to become actively involved in designing your own pain management plan – and to be creative about what you put into it.

- Pain is experienced in the brain. It is very real, but not some separate physical process signalling the severity of injury or trauma to the body. There are no 'pain nerves' which carry pain – only nerves which tell the brain there may be a problem.

- Chronic pain is made worse when our brains 'over-sensitise' the central and peripheral nervous systems, making us very aware of anything wrong but also potentially interpreting our chronic condition as life-threatening or capable of causing serious damage. Acute pain is very different and needs investigation and treatment as soon as possible.

- People used to think they could do little about pain until they were healed, except take drugs to ease its severity. We now know that's untrue and have physiological evidence explaining how thinking, feelings of security and risk, motivation and emotions affect pain perception.

- People experience pain in personal and individual ways, often related to their expectations, experience and outlook. See the Pain Management Wheel in Chapter 5.

- Becoming our own pain manager means understanding that our perceptions and thinking can influence our ability to cope and our resilience and can even influence our perceptions of pain level and intensity. But we know this works as a result of research and neuroscience rather than 'half-baked philosophy' or the 'power of positive thinking'.
- Self-managing pain isn't easy because there are many factors affecting motivation and resilience which are at work when you feel ill, become tired, stressed or depressed. Plans to control pain better need to address these issues too.

I hope this book will have helped you reassess and gain new ideas about your own pain management, although a book on its own is no substitute for the support of others – including friends, pain clinic groups and specialised charities. When you start to put your plan into action, remember the value of having someone to talk to, particularly during times of setback: someone who knows you and understands your situation. Try to get access to a pain clinic if your local hospital runs one; value your friends who can offer a helping hand; talk openly about what you are trying to achieve with your family and loved ones. And seek help from your doctor when you need it.

Support can also come from becoming a member of one of the national or local charities which specialise in your condition. It is useful to belong to a network of people who share your problems and are working positively to find ways of coping with the pain. It is important to have encouraging people to help you maintain what you learn about pain management, to help you think through the situation and to challenge your thinking. To tell you occasionally that you need to work at it a bit harder. As I said in the introduction, it isn't helpful for you to accept the patient role and adopt the outlook of an invalid.

The book is about taking back control of your pain – and, of course, your life. Being mobile and taking a full role in the life of your friends and family is an essential part of that. Be a bit tolerant about the technical bits in the book. They may need to be read a few times to see how our understanding about influencing/controlling pain has changed – but it's worth it. The most unappreciated part of our pain control system is the way our thoughts, emotions and the brain influence our nervous systems and vary the pain we experience.

Ultimately, the major task of pain management belongs to you. Use the book to think about what you need, what you'd like to try and who can help. Take small steps to begin your journey and give yourself credit for achieving even small improvements. Good luck!

David

Further Reading

These books are currently in print and should be available from most bookshops. They are useful for the general reader and don't require previous reading nor clinical experience.

Managing Pain Before It Manages You. (3rd edn). Margaret Caudill. New York: Guilford Press, 2008. ISBN: 9781593859824

Explain Pain. David S. Butler and G. Lorimer Moseley. Adelaide: Noigroup Publications, 2003. ISBN: 9780975091005

Overcoming Chronic Pain: A Self-Help Guide Using Cognitive Behavioural Techniques. Frances Cole et al. London: Constable and Robinson, 2010. ISBN: 9781841199702

Authentic Happiness. Martin Seligman. London: Nicholas Brealy Publishing, 2017. ISBN: 9781857886771

The Mindful Way through Depression: Freeing Yourself from Chronic Unhappiness. Mark Williams et al. New York: Guilford Press, 2007. ISBN: 9781593851286

British Pain Society publications are also a valuable source of information on everything from taking opioids to understanding long-term pain: www.britishpainsociety.org/british-pain-society-publications/patient-publications

The British Pain Society also provides a useful list of websites for regional, national and international organisations: www.britishpainsociety.org/useful-addresses

Finally, the author's website contains a range of free publications to read online: www.cog-escape-net.org.uk/resources

Endnotes

1   A. Nilakantan, J. Younger, A. Aron, and S. Mackey, 'Preoccupa-
     tion in an early-romantic relationship predicts pain relief', *Pain
     Medicine*, Vol. 15, no. 6 (June 2014): 947–53.

2   G.L. Moseley, T.J. Parsons, and C. Spence, 'Visual distortion of
     a limb modulates pain and swelling', *Current Biology*, Vol. 18,
     no. 22 (November 2008): 355–68.

3   M. Höfle, M. Hauck, A.K. Engel, and D. Senkowski, 'Viewing
     a needle pricking a hand that you perceive as yours enhances
     unpleasantness of pain', *PAIN*, Vol. 153, no. 5 (May 2012).

4   R. Severeijns, J.W. Vlaeyen, M.A. van den Hout, and W.E.
     Weber, 'Pain Catastrophizing Predicts Pain Intensity, Disability,
     and Psychological Distress Independent of the Level of Phys-
     ical Impairment', *The Clinical Journal of Pain*, Vol. 17, no. 2
     (June 2001): 165–72.

5   S.M. Jay, M. Ozolins, C.H. Elliott, and S. Caldwell, 'Assess-
     ment of children's distress during painful medical procedures',
     Health Psychology, Vol. 2, no. 2 (1983): 133–47.

6   'Mindfulness Report 2010', Mental Health Foundation: 42–8.
     https://www.mentalhealth.org.uk/publications/be-mindful-
     report

7   L. Torma, 'Fibromyalgia Pain and Physical Function: The influ-
     ence of resilience', *Scholar Archive*, 485 (2010): 56–9. https://
     digitalcommons.ohsu.edu/etd/485

8   H. Buttle, 'Attention and Working Memory in Mindfulness-
     Meditation Practices', *Journal of Mind and Behavior*, Vol. 32,
     no. 2 (spring 2011): 123–34.

9 A.P. Jha, J. Krompinger, and M.J. Baime, 'Mindfulness Training Modifies Subsystems of Attention', *Cognitive, Affective, & Behavioural Neuroscience*, Vol. 7, no. 2 (June 2007): 109–19.

10 J.M. Williams et al., 'Mindfulness-Based Cognitive Therapy for Preventing Relapse in Recurrent Depression: A Randomized Dismantling Trial', *Journal of Consulting and Clinical Psychology*, Vol. 82, no. 2 (April 2014): 275–86.

11 K. Neff and C. Germer, 'Self-Compassion and Psychological Well-Being', in *The Oxford Handbook of Compassion Science*, ed. E.M. Seppälä et al. (Oxford: Oxford University Press, 2017), 374–6.

12 A good source of information about the effects of inflammation can be found at: www.ouh.nhs.uk/oxparc/information/diagnoses/inflammatory-diseases.aspx

   Pain researchers have also been exploring how inflammation can be managed better; for further information, see the *British Journal of Anaesthesia*, Vol. 87, issue 1. https://doi.org/10.1093/bja/87.1.3

13 A guide to foods which can help minimise negative effects of inflammation can be found at: https://www.cog-escape-net.org.uk/resources